DOPING IN SPORTS

DOPING IN SPORTS

CHRISTOPHER N. BURNS
EDITOR

Nova Science Publishers, Inc.
New York

Copyright © 2006 by Nova Science Publishers, Inc.

All rights reserved. No part of this book may be reproduced, stored in a retrieval system or transmitted in any form or by any means: electronic, electrostatic, magnetic, tape, mechanical photocopying, recording or otherwise without the written permission of the Publisher.

For permission to use material from this book please contact us:
Telephone 631-231-7269; Fax 631-231-8175
Web Site: http://www.novapublishers.com

NOTICE TO THE READER

The Publisher has taken reasonable care in the preparation of this book, but makes no expressed or implied warranty of any kind and assumes no responsibility for any errors or omissions. No liability is assumed for incidental or consequential damages in connection with or arising out of information contained in this book. The Publisher shall not be liable for any special, consequential, or exemplary damages resulting, in whole or in part, from the readers' use of, or reliance upon, this material.

This publication is designed to provide accurate and authoritative information with regard to the subject matter covered herein. It is sold with the clear understanding that the Publisher is not engaged in rendering legal or any other professional services. If legal or any other expert assistance is required, the services of a competent person should be sought. FROM A DECLARATION OF PARTICIPANTS JOINTLY ADOPTED BY A COMMITTEE OF THE AMERICAN BAR ASSOCIATION AND A COMMITTEE OF PUBLISHERS.

LIBRARY OF CONGRESS CATALOGING-IN-PUBLICATION DATA
Available upon request

ISBN 1-59454-683-5

Published by Nova Science Publishers, Inc. ✣*New York*

CONTENTS

Preface		vii
Chapter 1	Anti-Doping Policies: The Olympics and Selected Professional Sports *L. Elaine Halchin*	1
Chapter 2	Federally Mandated Random Drug Testing in Professional Athletics: Constitutional Issues *Charles V. Dale*	37
Chapter 3	Drug Testing in Sports: Proposed Legislation *Nathan Brooks*	47
Chapter 4	Dietary Supplements: Ephedra *Donna V. Porter*	55
Index		79

PREFACE

The use of performance-enhancing substances by athletes has a long history, predating the ancient Greek Olympiads. Concern about this practice was manifested in the 20th century by, in the case of the Olympics, the creation of anti-doping organizations, and the adoption of anti-doping policies by these organizations and professional sports leagues in the United States. Leading the way was the International Olympic Committee (IOC), which implemented testing in 1968 at the Olympic Games in Grenoble, France, and Mexico City, Mexico. The National Basketball Association (NBA) and the National Football League (NFL) followed suit in the 1980s. Major League Baseball implemented an anti-drug policy in 2003. This report compares current anti-doping policies for performance enhancing substances among the Olympic movement and three professional sports — Major League Baseball, the NBA, and the NFL. Details associated with each of the selected group's policy are presented.

In: Doping in Sports
Editor: C. N. Burns, pp. 1-36

ISBN 1-59454-683-5
© 2006 Nova Science Publishers, Inc.

Chapter 1

ANTI-DOPING POLICIES: THE OLYMPICS AND SELECTED PROFESSIONAL SPORTS*

L. Elaine Halchin
Analyst in American National Government Government and Finance Division

SUMMARY

The use of performance-enhancing substances by athletes has a long history, predating the ancient Greek Olympiads. Concern about this practice was manifested in the 20th century by, in the case of the Olympics, the creation of anti-doping organizations, and the adoption of anti-doping policies by these organizations and professional sports leagues in the United States. Leading the way was the International Olympic Committee (IOC), which implemented testing in 1968 at the Olympic Games in Grenoble, France, and Mexico City, Mexico. The National Basketball Association (NBA) and the National Football League (NFL) followed suit in the 1980s. Major League Baseball implemented an anti-drug policy in 2003.

This report compares current anti-doping policies for performance enhancing substances among the Olympic movement and three professional sports — Major League Baseball, the NBA, and the

---

* Excerpted from CRS Report RL32894, dated April 29, 2005.

NFL. Details associated with each of the selected group's policy are presented in **Table 1**. The report also presents elements of what have been identified as model anti-doping policies and (in the appendix) provides a comparison of Major League Baseball's former and current anti-doping policies **(Table 2)** and a glossary of related terms.

In general, the report indicates that the anti-doping policies for the Olympic movement are more independent of the sports they regulate than are the policies of Major League Baseball, the NBA, and the NFL, both in the manner in which they are established and in the entities responsible for their implementation. For example, the World Anti-Doping Agency (WADA) unilaterally established the anti-doping policy for Olympic athletes, whereas the professional sports leagues' policies are the result of negotiations with their respective players associations. The Olympic movement also maintains the most comprehensive list of prohibited substances and methods, and provides sanctions that are more strict than in the professional sports. For example, the Olympic standard provides a two-year ban for a first violation, whereas Major League Baseball imposes a 10-day suspension without pay for a first violation. Also, Olympic athletes and NFL players are responsible for what is in their bodies, but neither Major League Baseball nor the NBA addresses this subject.

Direct comparison of these sports is sometimes difficult because the policies use different terminology or make reference to other standards. The policies are also constantly changing in response to the development of new substances that are sometimes designed to avoid detection. In some cases, the policies prohibit certain substances for which tests are not available in order to inform athletes about harmful substances. However, in other cases, tests and sanctions are not provided for substances for which tests are available. For example, except for "reasonable cause" testing, Major League Baseball's policy provides for testing and sanctions only with regard to steroids — not other substances prohibited in the league's policy.

This report will be updated as anti-doping policies change and elements of those policies become clearer.

ANTI-DOPING POLICIES

While the use of drugs and other substances — such as alcohol, ether, strychnine, anabolic steroids, stimulants, and hallucinogenic mushrooms —

as a means of improving athletic performance has a lengthy history, predating the ancient Greek Olympiads, condemnation of the practice did not surface until the early 20th century.[1] In 1933, Dr. Otto Reiser commented that

> [t]he use of artificial means [*to improve performance*] has long been considered wholly incompatible with the spirit of sport and has therefore been condemned. Nevertheless, we all know that this rule is continually being broken, and that sportive competitions are often more a matter of doping than of training. It is highly regrettable that those who are in charge of supervising sport seem to lack the energy for the campaign against this evil, and that a lax, and fateful, attitude is spreading."[2]

Despite such concerns about the use of performance-enhancing substances (PES) by athletes, anti-doping policies for the Olympic movement and major professional sports leagues in the United States were not drafted until the latter part of the 20th century.

- The International Olympic Committee (IOC) implemented testing in 1968, at the Olympic Games in Grenoble, France, and Mexico City, Mexico. Anabolic steroids were added by the IOC to its list of prohibited substances in 1976.[3]
- The National Football League (NFL) followed suit, in 1982, when it began to test players, although testing for anabolic steroids did not begin until 1987.[4] The NFL and the players association have updated their anti-doping policy several times since then. In testimony he presented at a congressional hearing in April 2005, the Commissioner of the NFL stated that the league and the players association recently had agreed to several changes to their policy and that the changes will take effect in 2005.[5] However, because these changes have not been formally published yet, this report treats their last public policy as the current policy.
- The National Basketball Association's (NBA) first anti-doping policy was issued in 1983, and it has been updated several times.[6]
- Major League Baseball implemented an anti-doping policy in 2003. Apparently in response to public pressure, Major League Baseball and the Major League Baseball Players Association (MLBPA) reopened the collective bargaining agreement in 2005 and updated the policy. Although the 2005 policy has not been ratified yet by the

players, it appears to be in effect and is treated in this report as the current policy.

This report compares current anti-doping policies among the Olympic movement and three professional sports — Major League Baseball, the NBA, and the NFL.[7] However, this issue clearly transcends these three leagues and the Olympics, and affects other professional sports and amateur athletics. Details associated with each of the selected group's policy are presented in **Table 1**. Although the antidoping policies in this report sometimes include so-called "recreational" drugs such as cocaine and marijuana, this report generally focuses on performance-enhancing substances. Also, it is important to emphasize that the descriptions and comparisons made here reflect the different sports' anti-doping *policies*, not their *implementation*. In addition, this report presents elements of what have been identified as model antidoping policies and, in the appendix, provides a comparison of Major League Baseball's former and current anti-doping policies (**Table 2**) and a glossary of related terms.

Olympic Policies More Independent of Regulated Sports

In general, this report indicates that the anti-doping policies for the Olympic movement are more independent of the sports they regulate than are the policies of Major League Baseball, the NBA, and the NFL, both in the manner in which they are established and in the entities responsible for their implementation. For example, the anti-doping policies of the professional sports leagues are established through a collective bargaining process between a players association and the applicable league, both of which benefit from professional players' performances. These policies also are administered by entities selected by the players associations and the leagues (for example, the members of baseball's Health Policy Advisory Committee are selected by Major League Baseball and the Major League Baseball Players Association). By contrast, in the Olympic movement, the World Anti-Doping Agency (WADA) unilaterally established the anti-doping policy and has no vested interested in the athletes' performances. The organization which administers this policy for U.S. Olympic athletes, the U.S. Anti-Doping Agency (USADA), also is independent of athletes and the organization that supports these athletes, the USOC.[8]

Table 1. Comparison of Selected Features of Anti-Doping Policies

	Olympic Movement	Major League Baseball MLB) and Major League Baseball Players Association (MLBPA) (2005 policy)a	National Basketball Association (NBA) and National Basketball Players Association (NBPA)	National Football League (NFL) and National Football League Players Association (NFLPA)
— What organization or individual is responsible for administering the anti-doping policy?	— U.S. Anti-Doping Agency (for American athletes).	— Health Policy Advisory Committee (HPAC).	— Medical director.	— NFL Advisor on Anabolic Steroids and Related Substances.
— Is the organization or individual independent from the sponsoring organization(s)?	—Yes.	— No. MLB and MLBPA each select two members of the HPAC.	— No. The medical director is selected jointly by the NBA and NBPA.	— No. The program is conducted under the auspices of the NFL Management Council, and it appears that the Advisor is an employee of the NFL.b
Is testing conducted offseason (or out of competition, for the Olympics)?	Yes.	Yes.	No, except possibly for "reasonable cause" testing.c	Yes.
Is an athlete responsible for prohibited substances found in his or her body?	Yes.	Subject is not addressed in the policy.	Subject is not addressed in the policy.	Yes.
Does the responsible organization test athletes for all prohibited substances?	No.f	No (steroids only).g	Yes.f	No.f

Table 1. Comparison of Selected Features of Anti-Doping Policies (Continued)

	Olympic Movement	Major League Baseball MLB and Major League Baseball Players Association (MLBPA) (2005 policy)a	National Basketball Association (NBA) and National Basketball Players Association (NBPA)	National Football League (NFL) and National Football League Players Association (NFLPA)
Does the anti-doping policy prohibit:[d]				
— Steroids	— Yes.	— Yes.	— Yes.	— Yes.
— Hormones and related substances	— Yes.	— Yes.[h]	— No.	— Yes.[i]
— Beta-2 agonists	— Yes.	— Unclear.[j]	— No.	— Yes.
— Agents with antiestrogenic activity	— Yes.	— Unclear.[k]	— No.	— No.
— Diuretics and other masking agents	— Yes.	— Unclear.[l]	— Unclear.[m]	— Yes.
— Enhancement of oxygen transfer	— Yes.	— No.	— No.	— No.
— Chemical and physical manipulation	— Yes.	— Unclear.[l]	— Unclear.[m]	— Yes.
— Gene doping	— Yes.	— No.	— No.	— No.
— Stimulants	— Yes.	— Unknown, except for ephedra, which is prohibited but not tested.[n]	— Yes, but only amphetamine and its analogues.	— Yes.
— Glucocorticosteroids	— Yes, but only in competition.	— Unclear.[o]	— No.	— No.
— Beta-blockers	— Yes, but only for certain sports.	— Unclear.[p]	— No.	— No.

Table 1. Comparison of Selected Features of Anti-Doping Policies (Continued)

	Olympic Movement	Major League Baseball MLB and Major League Baseball Players Association (MLBPA) (2005 policy)a	National Basketball Association (NBA) and National Basketball Players Association (NBPA)	National Football League (NFL) and National Football League Players Association (NFLPA)
What laboratory tests the samples?	WADA-accredited laboratories or as otherwise approved by WADA.	Subject is not addressed in the policy, but MLB has indicated that testing is conducted at a WADA accredited laboratory in Montreal.[q]	Laboratories are selected by the medical director, approved by the NBA and NBPA, and certified by the International Olympic Committee and/or the College of American Pathologists (for steroids), or the Substance Abuse and Mental Health Services Administration (for substances other than steroids).[r]	Under the existing collective bargaining agreement, samples to be analyzed for prohibited substances are to be submitted to the UCLA Olympic Analytical Laboratory at the UCLA School of Medicine.[s]
Are sanctions applicable to all prohibited substances?	Yes.	No (steroids only).[t]	Yes.	Yes.[u]

Table 1. Comparison of Selected Features of Anti-Doping Policies (Continued)

	Olympic Movement	Major League Baseball MLB and Major League Baseball Players Association (MLBPA) (2005 policy)a	National Basketball Association (NBA) and National Basketball Players Association (NBPA)	National Football League (NFL) and National Football League Players Association (NFLPA)
What are the sanctions for testing positive?				
— First violation	— Two-year ban[v]	— Steroids: 10-day suspension without pay.	— Steroids: Five-game suspension and required to enter steroids program. Amphetamines: First-year player is dismissed from the NBA for one year and required to enter treatment program. A veteran player is dismissed from the NBA for a minimum of two years.[w]	— Suspended without pay for a minimum of four games.
— Second violation	— Lifetime ban.	— 30-day suspension without pay.	— Steroids: 10-game suspension and required to enter steroids program.	— Suspended without pay for a minimum of six games.
— Third violation	— Not applicable.	— 60-day suspension without pay.	— Steroids: 25-game suspension and required to enter steroids program.	— Suspended without pay for at least 12 months.
— Fourth violation	— Not applicable.	— One-year suspension without pay.	— Steroids: Same as third violation.	— Not addressed.
— Subsequent violation(s)	— Not applicable.	— MLB Commissioner imposes further discipline.	— Steroids: Same as third violation.	— Not addressed.

Table 1. Comparison of Selected Features of Anti-Doping Policies (Continued)

	Olympic Movement	Major League Baseball MLB and Major League Baseball Players Association (MLBPA) (2005 policy)a	National Basketball Association (NBA) and National Basketball Players Association (NBPA)	National Football League (NFL) and National Football League Players Association (NFLPA)
What types of specimens are collected and tested?	Blood or urine.	Urine.	Urine. However, the medical director has authority to determine the use of blood, breath, or other testing techniques.	Urine.

Sources: U.S. Anti-Doping Agency, *United States Anti-Doping Agency Protocol for Olympic Movement Testing*, revised Aug. 13, 2004, available at [http://www.usantidoping.org/files/active/what/protocol.pdf]; U.S. Anti-Doping Agency, "USADA Press Kit" Jan. 2005, available at [http://www.usantidoping.org/files/active/resources/press_kits/2005%20Fact%20Sheet.pdf]; World Anti-Doping Agency, *World Anti-Doping Code*, 2003, available at [http://www.wada-ama.org/rtecontent/document/code_v3.pdf]; World Anti-Doping Agency, *International Standard for Testing*, June 2003, available at [http://www.wada-ama.org/rtecontent/document/testing_v3_a.pdf]; World Anti-Doping Agency, *International Standard for Therapeutic Use Exemptions*, n.d., available at [http://www.wada-ama.org/rtecontent/document/international_standard.pdf]; World Anti-Doping Agency, *The 2005 Prohibited List, International Standard*, n.d., available at [http://www.wada-ama.org/rtecontent/document/list_book_2005_en.pdf]; Major League Baseball, *Major League Baseball's Joint Drug Prevention and Treatment Program*, n.d., available at [http://reform.house.gov/UploadedFiles/031705%20MLB%20Policy.pdf]; National Basketball Players Association, *NBPA Collective Bargaining Agreement*, n.d., available at [http://www.nbpa.com/cba]; National Football League, *National Football League Policy on Anabolic Steroids and Related Substances*, 2003 (as amended May 15, 2003).

Notes:

a. The policy negotiated by Major League Baseball and the players association that takes effect during the 2005 season has not yet been ratified by the players, but apparently it is in effect. An article issued by *MLB.com* stated that an outfielder for the Tampa Bay Devil Rays tested positive for steroid use and, as a result, was suspended for the 10 days. (Barry M. Bloom, "Rays' Sanchez Suspended for 10 Days," *MLB.com*, Apr. 3, 2005, available at [http://mlb.mlb.com/NASApp/mlb/mlb/news/mlbsearcharchive.jsp].

b. The NFL Management Council oversees policies that relate to players, including the collective bargaining agreement. The council reports to the Commissioner of the National Football League. (Information provided by telephone by the NFL Communications Department to the author on Apr. 18, 2005.)

c. Reasonable cause testing is conducted when the Independent Expert who has been selected by the NBA and the NBPA has determined "there is reasonable cause to believe that the player in question has been engaged in the use, possession, or distribution of a Prohibited Substance." (National Basketball Players Association, *NBPA Collective Bargaining Agreement*, n.d., available at [http://www.nbpa.com/cba], Sec. 5(a).)

d. The detail and extent of an anti-doping policy's list of prohibited substances and methods vary from organization to organization. One possible reason for variations among the lists is that some substances may benefit only athletes in certain sports. For example, beta-blockers, which decrease the heart rate and may aid in decreasing tremors or shaking, may be used by athletes who participate in sports that reward precision and accuracy, such as archery.

e. The use of the term "steroids" in this context refers to anabolic or anabolic androgenic steroids, substances which may help an athlete increase his or her muscle size and strength and recover more quickly from injury. The class of substances known as "steroids" includes other types of substances. See "anabolic androgenic steroids" and "steroids" in the glossary.

f. In some cases, accurate laboratory tests do not exist for certain prohibited substances or levels. In other cases, though (e.g., the NFL's policy on human growth hormone), tests are available to detect the prohibited substances but are not used. The NBA tests for all prohibited substances, but its list of such substances is shorter than the lists for the other sports.

g. The federal government has established five schedules of controlled substances. The following three criteria are used to determine on which schedule to place a substance or drug: its potential for abuse, whether the item has a currently accepted medical use in the United States, and the probability that abuse of the substance could lead to physical or psychological dependence. Schedule I includes substances and drugs that have a high potential for abuse, that currently have no accepted medical use in the United States, and that lack accepted safety for use under medical supervision. Substances and drugs listed on one of the remaining four schedules have currently accepted medical uses, and the potential for abuse and the probability that abuse could lead to physical or psychological dependence declines from Schedule II through Schedule IV. (21 U.S.C. § 812(a) and (b).) Major League Baseball's list of prohibited substances includes drugs of abuse (cocaine, LSD, marijuana, opiates, Ecstasy, GHB, PCP, ephedra, all drugs or substances listed on Schedule II, and all Schedule I drugs listed on Addendum B of the league's anti-doping policy) and all anabolic androgenic steroids listed on Schedule III. Section 3.B. of this policy explicitly excludes drugs of abuse from the testing program: "Except as set forth in Section 3.C. [reasonable cause testing], Players shall not be subject to testing for the use of any Drug of Abuse." (Major League Baseball, *Major League Baseball's Joint Drug Prevention and Treatment Program*, n.d., pp. 3 and 6, available at [http://reform.house.gov/UploadedFiles/ 031705%20MLB%20Policy.pdf].)

h. Human growth hormone (hGH) is on the list of prohibited substances, under the heading "steroids," but MLB does not test for it. In testimony offered during a House Committee on Government Reform hearing, Robert D. Manfred Jr., Executive Vice President, MLB, and Elliot J. Pellman, M.D., Medical Advisor to the Commissioner of Baseball, indicated that Major League Baseball does not test for human growth hormone (hGH). The rationale they offered was that no valid urine-based test exists. Mr. Manfred added: "Contrary to published reports, there is not an available, verified test for HGH, even with a blood sample." (U.S. Congress, House Committee on Government Reform, statements of Robert D. Manfred Jr., Executive Vice President, Major League Baseball, and Elliot J. Pellman, M.D., Medical Advisor the Commissioner of Baseball, unpublished hearing, 109th Cong., 1st sess., Mar. 17, 2005, available at [http://mlb.mlb.com/NASApp/mlb/news/press_releases/intro.jsp] and [http://reform.house.gov/Uploaded Files/Pellman%20Testimony.pdf].) It should be noted that the World Anti-Doping Agency tested athletes for hGH at the 2004 Athens Olympics, using a blood test that had been developed and validated in partnership with the IOC and USADA. (World Anti Doping Agency, "Minutes of the WADA Executive Committee Meeting," Nov. 20, 2004, p. 20, available at [http://www.wada-ama. org/en/dynamic.ch2?pageCategory_id=44].)

i. As an example of how the lists of prohibited substances vary from organization to organization, only human growth hormone, animal growth hormone, and human chorionic gonadotropin are included on the NFL's list of hormones. The WADA list includes several other hormones and related substances. (World Anti-Doping Agency, *International Standard for Testing*, June 2003, available at [http://www.wada-ama.org/rtecontent/document/testing_v3_a.pdf]).

j. The list of prohibited substances includes all of Schedule II and an extensive list of substances from Schedule I. It is unclear whether any substances known as "beta-2 agonists" are listed on either of these schedules. Efforts to obtain clarification on this matter from Major League Baseball or the players association are continuing.

k. The list of prohibited substances includes all of Schedule II and an extensive list of substances from Schedule I. It is unclear whether any substances known as agents with antiestrogenic activity are listed on either of these schedules. Efforts to obtain clarification on this matter from Major League Baseball or the players association are continuing.

l. Masking substances (and methods) are not identified on the list of prohibited substances, but the policy states: "Attempts to substitute, dilute, mask, or adulterate a specimen sample are considered a positive test result." (*Major League Baseball, Major League Baseball's Joint Drug Prevention and Treatment Program*, p. 6.)

m. Masking substances (and methods) are not identified on the list of prohibited substances. However, the policy states that "[if a player attempts to substitute, dilute, mask, or adulterate a specimen sample or in any other manner [alter] a test result," such activity or action will be considered a positive test. (National Basketball Players Association, *NBPA Collective Bargaining Agreement*, Sec. 4(c)(iv).)

n. The list of prohibited substances includes all of Schedule II and an extensive list of substances from Schedule I. It is unclear whether any substances known as stimulants are listed on either of these schedules. Efforts to obtain clarification on this matter from Major League Baseball or the players association are continuing. While ephedra is a prohibited substance, it is found on the "Drugs of Abuse" list, which means it is not included in regular testing of players. (*Major League Baseball, Major League Baseball's Joint Drug Prevention and Treatment Program*, p. 3.)

o. The list of prohibited substances includes all of Schedule II and an extensive list of substances from Schedule I. It is unclear whether any substances known as glucocorticosteroids are listed on either of these schedules. Efforts to obtain clarification on this matter from Major League Baseball or the players association are continuing.

p. The list of prohibited substances includes all of Schedule II and an extensive list of substances from Schedule I. It is unclear whether any substances known as beta-blockers are listed on either of these schedules. Efforts to obtain clarification on this matter from Major League Baseball or the players association are continuing.

q. Major League Baseball and the players association agreed, in spring 2004, to have all drug testing conducted by the Doping Control Laboratory at the INES-Instituted Armand-Flapper Research Center in Montreal. This is a WADA-accredited laboratory. (Major League Baseball, "MLB Drug-Testing Programs Move to Olympic-Certified Laboratories," May 11, 2004, available at [http://mlb.mlb.com/NASApp/mlb/content/printerfriendly/Mb/y2004/m05/d11/c740823.jsp].)

r. The Substance Abuse and Mental Health Services Administration is an agency within the Department of Health and Human Services.

s. This is a WADA-accredited laboratory.

t. This sanction is specific to Articles 2.1 (presence of a prohibited substance in an athlete's substance), 2.2 (use or attempted use of a prohibited substance or a prohibited method), and 2.6 (possession of prohibited substances and methods) in the WADA Code. For the list of sanctions imposed for other violations, see the WADA Code, pp. 27-35. An athlete who has been banned under the WADA Code has been declared ineligible. An athlete's status during eligibility is as follows: "No Person who has been declared ineligible may, during the period of ineligibility, participate in any capacity in a Competition or activity (other than authorized anti-doping education or rehabilitation programs) authorized or organized by a Signatory or Signatory's member organization" (p. 35). Signatories are those organizations that have signed and agreed to comply with the WADA Code and include "the International Olympic Committee, International Federations, International Paralympic Committee, National Olympic Committees, National Paralympic Committees, Major Event Organizations, National Anti-Doping Organizations, and WADA." (World Anti-Doping Agency, *World Anti-Doping Code*, 2003, available at [http://www.wada-ama.org/rtecontent/document/code_v3.pdf], pp. 35, 75.) For example, the list of organizations that have accepted the WADA Code includes the International Fencing Federation, International Swimming Federation, International Tennis Federation, and the International Wrestling Federation. (World Anti-Doping Agency, "List of Sports Organizations Who Have Accepted the Code," n.d., available at [http://www.wada-ama.org/en/print.asp?p=42255].)

u. It is unclear what sanction, if any, the NFL would impose on a player who uses masking agents or otherwise practices pharmacological, chemical or physical manipulation of a sample. Both masking agents and doping methods (that is, manipulation) are included on the list of prohibited substances. However, the policy states that "Any effort to substitute, dilute, or adulterate a specimen or to alter a test result may subject a player to more severe discipline than would have been imposed for a positive test." (National Football League, *National Football League Policy on Anabolic Steroids and Related Substances*, pp. 4, 11-12.) The use of the word "may" suggests that the NFL may exercise discretion when dealing with a player who has attempted to alter, or has altered, a test. The phrase "than would have been imposed for a positive test" suggests that the NFL does not treat test alteration the same as a positive laboratory test for a prohibited substance. Efforts to resolve this matter are ongoing.

v. Apparently, these sanctions apply only to positive tests for steroids. As noted above, testing for other substances and drugs prohibited by the league will not be done as part of its ongoing testing program (though players may be tested for these other substances when reasonable cause exists). Nevertheless, it bears noting that no sanctions are included for positive tests of other substances. The 2005 draft of Mb's anti-doping policy states that, for first through fourth violations, a fine may be levied in lieu of imposing a suspension. (Major League Baseball, *Major League Baseball's Joint Drug Prevention and Treatment Program*, n.d., pp. 11-12.) However, as reported in the *Washington Post* on Mar. 21, 2005, both parties (MB and MLBPA) have agreed to eliminate fines, leaving suspensions as the only sanction. ("Agreement Reached to Drop Fines," *Washington Post*, Mar. 21, 2005, p. D5.)

w. Apparently, the MBA's policy does not mention what, if any, penalties are imposed for subsequent violations involving the use of amphetamines.

A comparison of selected features of anti-doping policies shows, among other things, that the Olympic movement maintains the most comprehensive list of prohibited substances and methods. This may be due, at least in part, to the general understanding that some substances or drugs benefit only athletes in certain sports.[9] For example, a drug that slows down heart rate and reduces fine motor tremors would be more helpful to an archer than a basketball player. Another feature on which the Olympic movement and most professional sports leagues differ is whether an athlete is responsible for the substances discovered is in his or her body. In both the Olympics and the NFL, an athlete is responsible, but neither Major League Baseball nor the NBA addresses this subject in their written policies. Sanctions for testing positive also vary. The Olympic movement imposes the most stringent penalties: the first violation results in a two-year ban, and a second violation results in a lifetime ban from competition, as defined by WADA.[10] In contrast, according to Major League Baseball's current policy, a second violation results only in a 30-day suspension without pay.

Issues in Comparing Anti-Doping Policies

The structure and content of these sports' anti-doping policies vary in a number of ways, including the subjects covered in those policies, the extent of detail provided, and the language and terminology used to identify or describe prohibited substances. As a result, direct comparison of the policies is extremely difficult, and certain of their provisions may be subject to differing interpretations. Also, various contextual factors need to be considered when comparing the different sports' antidoping policies.

Identifying Prohibited Substances/Methods

It is sometimes difficult to determine which specific substances and methods are prohibited in an anti-doping policy. As a result, it is difficult to compare those policies. These difficulties can arise when different policies use different terminology, or when a policy refers to an associated statute or standard. For example, Major League Baseball's list of prohibited substances incorporates, by reference, several of the federal government's lists of controlled substances.[11] Examples of substance names found on one of the lists of controlled substances are clonitazene, etoxeridine, and the bacon. However, it is not clear whether any of these substances are beta-2 agonists, agents with antiestrogenic activity, glucocorticosteroids, or beta-blockers — classes of substances identified by WADA as performance-enhancing substances. Our efforts to obtain clarification from Major League Baseball or the players association on this and other matters are continuing.

Changing Nature of Policies

The nature of the problem of doping in sports has implications for the creation of lists of prohibited substances and testing policies. In some cases, performance enhancing substances being used by athletes may not appear on the lists of prohibited substances because sports officials are not aware of their existence or use. For example, in an effort to evade detection of steroid use, some athletes use designer steroids, which are described as follows:

> ... a designer or "new" steroid [is a substance that] has been chemically produced (synthesized in the laboratory)[and] that retains the anabolic properties desired for such a drug. At the same time the molecular structure ... is chemically altered so that the currently used steroid screening test will not ... [find the drug in an athlete's specimen] ....[12]

When it was created, tetrahydrogestrinone (THG) was a designer steroid. THG became known after a then-anonymous track and field coach in the United States provided a sample to USADA, which forwarded the sample to the UCLA Olympic Analytic Laboratory. Using this sample, the laboratory was able to identify the substance.[13] Because designer steroids are developed specifically to avoid detection, it is impossible for anti-doping organizations or sports leagues to include them on their lists of prohibited substances. Therefore, as new doping methods become known, anti-doping policies must be revisited from time to time to ensure they are up to date.

Some of the professional sports included in this report have recently changed their anti-doping policies. The NFL's April 2005 change reportedly tripled the number of times a player can be tested for steroids during the offseason, added to the league's list of prohibited substances, and allowed for retesting of a players' urine samples for designer steroids that may have been previously undetected.[14] A comparison of Major League Baseball's former and current policies (**Table 2** in the appendix) also shows several significant differences. Under the former policy, hormones may not have been prohibited; the list of sanctions allowed first-time offenders to be placed in a treatment program and permitted the imposition of a fine in lieu of a suspension without pay for second through fifth violations; and testing was not conducted during the off-season. The current policy prohibits the use of hormones, imposes a 10-day suspension without pay for a first violation and progressively longer suspensions without pay for subsequent violations, and testing is conducted during the off-season.

No Tests or Sanctions for Some Prohibited Substances

Anti-doping policies may not provide tests or sanctions for certain prohibited substances. In some cases, tests for those substances are available, but are not being used. For example, Section 3.B. of Major League Baseball's policy explicitly states that, except for "reasonable cause" testing, "Players shall not be subject to testing for the use of any Drug of Abuse."[15] Notably, included among the list of "drugs of abuse" is ephedra, which the league banned in the wake of a player's death in 2003. Therefore, although a test for ephedra is available, it is not currently included in the list of substances for which players are being tested. In fact, other than "reasonable cause" testing, Major League Baseball's policy does not provide for testing or sanctions for any prohibited substance other than steroids.[16]

In other cases, though, lists of prohibited substances may include known substances for which there are no laboratory tests, or, in the case of hormones and other substances that occur naturally in the human body, for which there is an insufficient amount of data to determine "what levels of ... hormones are abnormal or indicative of abuse and what levels are normal."[17] For example, natural hormones other than testosterone — such as human chorionic gonadotropin, insulin, and erythropoietin — may be found on lists of prohibited substances, but laboratory tests may not be available yet and what constitutes an abnormal level in the human body may not yet have been determined.

Nevertheless, including substances for which laboratory tests do not exist on a list of prohibited substances may serve an organization's purposes. For example, an organization may establish a list not only to alert athletes to doping tests but also to inform them about harmful substances. One of the purposes of the World Anti- Doping Program and the *World Anti-Doping Code* is "[t]o protect the Athletes' fundamental right to participate in doping-free sport and thus promote health, fairness and equality for Athletes worldwide ...."[18] Certain elements of the rationale for the *Code* may also have a bearing on the inclusion of substances for which tests are not yet available. These include, for example, "ethics, fair play and honesty .... health .... character and education .... respect for rules and laws .... respect for self and other participants ...."[19] The National Football League cites three reasons, including the health of players, for its concern about the use of prohibited substances:

[They] threaten the fairness and integrity of the athletic competition on the playing field .... [T]he League is concerned with the adverse health effects of steroid use. Although research is continuing, steroid use has been linked to a number of physiological, psychological, orthopedic, reproductive, and other serious health problems .... [T]he use of Prohibited Substances by NFL players sends the wrong message to young people who may be tempted to use them.[20]

Thus, it appears that these two organizations (WADA and the NFL), and possibly others as well, recognize that the value of an anti-doping program or policy extends beyond testing to include messages about harmful substances and how they might undermine other aspects of athletic competition.

Comparison of Olympic Movement, Major League Baseball, NBA, and NFL Anti-Doping Policies

Table 1 below compares specific elements of the anti-doping policies of the Olympic movement, Major League Baseball, the NBA, and the NFL. Those elements include which organizations administer the policies, the substances and methods prohibited, and the sanctions for testing positive for a prohibited substance. In many cases, reference to an associated footnote is needed to understand particular elements of a sport's policy.

ELEMENTS OF MODEL ANTI-DOPING POLICIES

Experts in the field of drug testing and policy have described what they believe to be the requisite elements of an effective anti-doping policy. For example, speaking at a Senate committee hearing in 2004, the Chief Executive Officer of USADA said such a policy:

> ... begins with a sample collection plan that includes appropriately timed, yearround, no-advance-notice testing. The plan must provide for the collection of samples at the time that athletes most benefit from doping and must be flexible and responsive to evolving doping techniques.
> ... must be built around a comprehensive list of categories of prohibited substances and methods .... programs must incorporate sufficient

flexibility to deal with the creation and use of 'designer drugs' .... Therefore, the continued dedication of resources to the testing laboratories that are charged with developing and validating testing methods for this wide array of substances is an important aspect of deterrence.

... also combines defined sanctions of sufficient magnitude to deter drug use with a fair means of imposing such sanctions .... Significantly, while USADA believes the privacy rights of individuals accused of a doping violation must be respected, no individual's right should outweigh the rights of all athletes to compete in clean sport and to be assured that those who break the rules are appropriately sanctioned. ...

[provides for] the education of athletes as to why healthy competition is important and why taking the uninformed health risks associated with prohibited substances is a bad choice. The achievements in sports, like the achievements in life, should be the result of hard work, commitment, and dedication.

... must devote significant resources to research for the detection of new doping substances and techniques and the pursuit of scientific excellence in doping control.[21]

Similarly, General Barry R. McCaffrey, U.S. Army (ret.), then-Director, Office of National Drug Control Policy, appeared at a Senate hearing in 1999 and stated that, with regard to international competition, the agency was focused on achieving these principles:

- A truly independent and accountable international anti-doping agency;
- Testing on a 365-day-a-year, no notice basis;
- No statute of limitations — whenever evidence becomes available that an athlete cheated by doping, the athlete will be stripped of his or her honors;
- Deterrence through the preservation of samples for at least 10 years — while a dishonest athlete may be able to defeat today's drug test, he or she has no way to know what will be detectable through tomorrow's scientific advances; and,
- Advanced research to end the present cat-and-mouse game of doping by closing the loopholes created by gaps in science.[22]

Conclusion

Combining elements of Madden's and McCaffrey's plans, such as a wellthought- out sample collection plan and a comprehensive list of prohibited substances, could result in an anti-doping program that would increase the probability of catching athletes who use prohibited substances, which, in turn, might also increase athletes' perceived risk of being caught. For example, requiring that samples be preserved for at least 10 years could aid in identifying athletes who have used performanceenhancing substances that were undetectable previously. As the investigation of the Bay Area Laboratory Co-Operative (BALCO) has shown, it is possible for individuals to develop what are known as designer steroids — substances that are advertised as providing effects similar to steroids, but are not identifiable by conventional laboratory tests.[23] A 10-year (or longer) retention period could help in closing this gap, particularly if it is accompanied by an aggressive research program aimed at detecting, and developing tests for, previously unknown substances. Also, imposing sanctions of sufficient magnitude and providing an education program on health risks could help to counterbalance incentives that might prompt athletes to use prohibited substances. Finally, establishment of an independent agency to manage testing, education, and research appears to be vital to a successful anti-doping program. It would seem desirable to place these functions in an organization independent from the organization that is responsible for supporting or employing athletes and that benefits directly, or even indirectly, from their performances.

While the anti-doping initiative of the Olympic movement includes many of these elements, it is uncertain whether major professional sports leagues in the United States, such as Major League Baseball and the NBA and NFL, are in a position to take similar steps. Public pressure and congressional interest may have played a role in prompting Major League Baseball and the players association to reopen their collective bargaining agreement in 2005 and modify the league's antidoping policy. One notable outcome was a change in the sanctions imposed on players caught using steroids.

APPENDIX

Table 2. Comparison of Selected Features of Major League Baseball's 2003-2004 Policy and 2005 Policy

	Major League Baseball MB) 2003-2004 Policy	Major League Baseball (MB) 2005 Policy (draft)a
— What organization or individual is responsible for administering the antidoping policy?	— Health Policy Advisory Committee (HPAC).	— HPAC.
— Is the organization or individual independent from the sponsoring organization(s)?	— No. Major League Baseball and the Major League Baseball Players Association each select two members of the HPAC.	— No.
Are athletes tested for all prohibited substances?	No.[f]	No.[f]
Does the anti-doping policy prohibit:		
— Steroidse	— Yes.	— Yes.
— Hormones and related substances	— Unclear.[l]	— Yes.[f]
— Beta-2 agonists	— Unclear.[l]	— Unclear.[l]
— Agents with antiestrogenic activity	— Unclear[l]	— Unclear.[l]
— Diuretics and other masking agents	— Yes.[i]	— Yes.[i]
— Enhancement of oxygen transfer	— No.	— No.
— Chemical and physical manipulation	— Yes.[i]	— Yes.[i]
— Gene doping	— No.	— No.
— Stimulants	— Unclear.[k]	— Unclear, except for ephedra, which is prohibited but not tested.[n,l]
— Glucocorticosteroids	— Unclear.[m]	— Unclear.[m]
Is a player responsible for what is in his body?	Unclear.[l]	No.
What laboratory tests the samples?	Subject is not addressed in the policy.	Subject is not addressed in the policy, but MB has indicated that testing is conducted at a WADAaccredited laboratory in Montreal.[q]

Table 2. Continued

	Major League Baseball MB) 2003-2004 Policy	Major League Baseball (MB) 2005 Policy (draft)a
Are sanctions applicable to all prohibited substances?	No.[f]	No.[f]
What are the sanctions for testing positive for steroids?		
— First violation	— Played placed on clinical track (treatment program).	— 10-day suspension without pay.[q]
— Second violation	— 15-day suspension without pay or a maximum fine of $10,000.	— 30-day suspension without pay.
— Third violation	— 25-day suspension without pay or a maximum fine of $25,000.	— 60-day suspension without pay.
— Fourth violation	— 50-day suspension without pay or a maximum fine of $50,000.	— One-year suspension without pay.
— Fifth violation	— One-year suspension without pay or a maximum fine of $100,000.	— MB Commissioner imposes further discipline.
Is testing conducted during the off-season?	No.	Yes
What types of specimens are collected and tested?	Urine.	Urine.

Sources: Major League Baseball, *Major League Baseball's Joint Drug Prevention and Treatment Program*, n.d., p. 6, available at [http://reform.house.gov/UploadedFiles/031705%20MLB%20Policy. pdf]; Major League Baseball and Major League Baseball Players Association, *2003-2006 Basic Agreement*, n.d., available at [http://us.i1.yimg.com/ us.yimg.com/i/spo /mlbpa/mlbpa_cba.pdf].

Notes:

[a.] The policy negotiated by Major League Baseball and the players association that takes effect during the 2005 season has not yet been ratified by the players, but apparently it is in effect. An article issued by *MLB.com* stated that an outfielder for the Tampa Bay Devil Rays tested positive for steroid use and, as a result, was suspended for the 10 days. (Barry M. Bloom, "Rays' Sanchez Suspended for 10 Days," *MLB.com*, Apr. 3, 2005, available at [http://mlb.mlb.com/NASApp/ mlb/mlb/news/mlb_ search_archive.jsp].

[b.] The federal government has established five schedules of controlled substances. The following three criteria are used to determine on which schedule to place a substance or drug: its potential for abuse, whether the item has a currently accepted medical use in the United States, and the probability that abuse of the substance could lead to physical or psychological dependence. Schedule I includes substances and drugs that have a high potential for abuse, that currently have no accepted medical use in the United States, and that lack accepted safety for use under medical supervision. Substances and drugs listed on one of the remaining four schedules have currently accepted medical uses, and the potential for abuse and the probability that abuse could lead to physical or psychological dependence declines from Schedule II through Schedule IV. (21 U.S.C. § 812(a) and (b).) Major League Baseball's list of prohibited substances includes drugs of abuse (cocaine, LSD, marijuana, opiates, Ecstasy, GHB, PCP, all drugs or substances listed on Schedule II, and all Schedule I drugs listed on Addendum C of the league's anti-doping policy) and all anabolic androgenic steroids listed on Schedule III. Section 3.C. of this policy explicitly excludes drugs of abuse from the testing program: "Except as set forth in Section 3.D. [reasonable cause testing], Players shall not be subject to either Survey or Program Testing for the use of any Drug of Abuse." (Major League Baseball and Major League Baseball Players Association, *2003-2006 Basic Agreement*, n.d., pp. 159-160, 163, available online at [http://us.i1.yimg.com/us.yimg.com/i/spo /mlbpa/mlbpa_cba.pdf].)

c. The federal government has established five schedules of controlled substances. The following three criteria are used to determine on which schedule to place a substance or drug: its potential for abuse, whether the item has a currently accepted medical use in the United States, and the probability that abuse of the substance could lead to physical or psychological dependence. Schedule I includes substances and drugs that have a high potential for abuse, that currently have no accepted medical use in the United States, and that lack accepted safety for use under medical supervision. Substances and drugs listed on one of the remaining four schedules have currently accepted medical uses, and the potential for abuse and the probability that abuse could lead to physical or psychological dependence declines from Schedule II through Schedule IV. (21 U.S.C. § 812(a) and (b).) Major League Baseball's list of prohibited substances includes drugs of abuse (cocaine, LSD, marijuana, opiates, Ecstasy, GHB, PCP, ephedra, all drugs or substances listed on Schedule II, and all Schedule I drugs listed on Addendum B of the league's anti-doping policy) and all anabolic androgenic steroids listed on Schedule III. Section 3.B. of this policy explicitly excludes drugs of abuse from the testing program: "Except as set forth in Section 3.C. [reasonable cause testing], Players shall not be subject to testing for the use of any Drug of Abuse." (Major League Baseball, *Major League Baseball's Joint Drug Prevention and Treatment*

Program, n.d., pp. 3 and 6, available at [http://reform.house.gov/Uploaded Files/ 031705%20MLB%20Policy.pdf].)

d. The use of the term "steroids" in this context refers to anabolic or anabolic androgenic steroids, substances which may help an athlete increase his or her muscle size and strength and re cover more quickly from injury. The class of substances known as "steroids" includes other types of substances. See "anabolic androgenic steroids" and "steroids" in the glossary.

e. The list of prohibited substances includes all of Schedule II and an extensive list of substances from Schedule I. It is unclear whether any substances known as "hormones" are listed on either of these schedules. Efforts to obtain clarification on this matter from Major League Baseball or the players association are continuing.

f. Human growth hormone (hGH) is on the list of prohibited substances, under the heading "steroids," but MB does not test for it. In testimony offered during a House Committee on Government Reform hearing, Robert D. Manfred Jr., Executive Vice President, MB, and Elliot J. Pellman, M.D., Medical Advisor to the Commissioner of Baseball, indicated that Major League Baseball does not test for human growth hormone (hGH). The rationale they offered was that no valid urine-based test exists. Mr. Manfred added: "Contrary to published reports, there is not an available, verified test for HGH, even with a blood sample." (U.S. Congress, House Committee on Government Reform, statements of Robert D. Manfred Jr., Executive Vice President, Major League Baseball, and Elliot J. Pellman, M.D., Medical Advisor to the Commissioner of Baseball, unpublished hearing, 109th Cong., 1st sess., Mar. 17, 2005, available online at [http://mlb.mlb.com/NASApp/mlb/news/press_releases/intro.jsp] and [http://reform.house.gov/UploadedFiles/Pellman%20Testimony.pdf].) It should be noted that the World Anti-Doping Agency tested athletes for hGH at the 2004 Athens Olympics, using a blood test that had been developed and validated in partnership with the IOC and USADA. (World Anti Doping Agency, "Minutes of the WADA Executive Committee Meeting," Nov. 20, 2004, p. 20, at [http://www.wada-ama.org/en/dynamic.ch2?pageCategory_id=44].)

g. The list of prohibited substances includes all of Schedule II and an extensive list of substances from Schedule I. It is unclear whether any substances known as "beta-2 agonists" are listed on either of these schedules. Efforts to obtain clarification on this matter from Major League Baseball or the players association are continuing.

h. The list of prohibited substances includes all of Schedule II and an extensive list of substances from Schedule I. It is unclear whether any substances known as "agents with anti-estrogenic activity" are listed on either of these schedules. Efforts to obtain clarification on this matter from Major League Baseball or the players association are continuing.

i. Masking substances (and methods) are not identified on the list of prohibited substances, but the policy states that any test will be considered "positive" if a player "attempts to substitute, dilute, mask, or adulterate a specimen sample or in any other manner alter a test." (Major League Baseball, *2003-2006 Basic Agreement*, p. 164.)

j. Masking substances (and methods) are not identified on the list of prohibited substances, but the policy states: "Attempts to substitute, dilute, mask, or adulterate a specimen sample are considered a positive test result." (Major League Baseball, *Major League Baseball's Joint Drug Prevention and Treatment Program*, p. 6.)

k. The list of prohibited substances includes all of Schedule II and an extensive list of substances from Schedule I. It is unclear whether any substances known as "stimulants" are listed on either of these schedules. Efforts to obtain clarification on this matter from Major League Baseball or the players association are continuing.

l. Ephedra is a prohibited substance, but it is not included in regular testing of players. (Major League Baseball, *Major League Baseball's Joint Drug Prevention and Treatment Program*, p. 3.) See footnote c. above.

m. The list of prohibited substances includes all of Schedule II and an extensive list of substances from Schedule I. It is unclear whether any substances known as "glucocorticosteroids" are listed on either of these schedules. Efforts to obtain clarification on this matter from Major League Baseball or the players association are continuing.

n. Absent an explicit statement about a player's responsibility for what is in his body, the following excerpt suggests that, depending upon the circumstances, a player's claim that a positive test resulted from a contaminated over-the-counter supplement could have been valid : "If ... a Player tests positive in the initial test for a Steroid and such positive test cannot be a result of a Player taking an over-the-counter supplement, the initial test shall be considered a positive result regardless of the outcome of the follow-up test."(Major League Baseball and Major League Baseball Players Association, *2003-2006 Basic Agreement*, p. 162.)

o. Major League Baseball and the players association agreed, in spring 2004, to have all drug testing under the *MB Joint Drug Prevention and Testing Program* conducted by the Doping Control Laboratory at the INRS-Instituted Armand-Flapper Research Center in Montreal. This is a WADA-accredited laboratory. (Major League Baseball, "MB Drug-Testing Programs Move to Olympic-Certified Laboratories," May 11, 2004, available at [http://mlb.mlb.com/NASApp/ mlb/content/printer_friendly/ mlb/y2004/m05/d11/c740823.jsp].)

p. Apparently, sanctions apply only to positive tests for steroids. As noted above, testing for other substances and drugs prohibited by the league will not be done as part of its ongoing testing program. Though players may be tested for these other substances when reasonable cause exists for doing so, no sanctions are included for positive tests of other substances.

q. The 2005 draft of MLB's anti-doping policy states that, for first through fourth violations, a fine may be levied in lieu of imposing a suspension. (Major League Baseball, *Major League Baseball's Joint Drug Prevention and Treatment Program*, n.d., pp. 11-12.) However, as reported in the *Washington Post* on Mar. 21, 2005, both parties (MB and MLBPA) have agreed to eliminate fines, leaving suspensions as the only sanction. ("Agreement Reached to Drop Fines," *Washington Post*, Mar. 21, 2005, p. D5.)

GLOSSARY

Agents with anti-estrogenic activity — An agent with anti-estrogenic activity blocks the conversion of testosterone to estrogens (female hormones), or prevents or minimizes the body's response to estrogens present in the body. A male athlete who uses steroids may ingest an agent with anti-estrogen activity to help mitigate against breast development resulting from steroid use.[24]

Anabolic androgenic steroids — "Anabolic-androgenic steroids [AAS] are synthetic derivatives of testosterone .... Testosterone itself is not effective when taken orally or by injection, because it is susceptible to relatively rapid breakdown by the liver. The chemical structure of testosterone has been modified by pharmaceutical companies and pharmacologists to surmount this problem."[25] "'Anabolic' refers to muscle-building, and 'androgenic' refers to increased masculine characteristics.[26] Using steroids may help an individual increase his or her muscle size and strength and recover more quickly from injury."[27] Also see "Steroids."

Analogues (analogs) — "[S]ubstances derived from the modification or alteration of the chemical structure of another substance while retaining a similar pharmacological effect."[28] For example, the chemical structure of a steroid analogue would differ from the structure of a steroid, but it would promote the development of muscle.

Beta-2 agonists — "Beta-agonists are bronchodilator medicines that open airways by relaxing the muscles around the airways that tighten during an asthma attack."[29] Some beta-2 agonists, when taken into the bloodstream, may help to increase "skeletal muscle mass and decrease body fat."[30]

Beta-blockers — "Beta-blockers are commonly used for heart disease to lower blood pressure and decrease the heart rate, and may be used to decrease fine motor tremor.[31] Athletes may use beta-blockers illegally to try to stop their hands and bodies from shaking while competing in precision sports that require accuracy, a calm state and/or a steady hand."[32]

Diuretics — "Diuretics remove the excess water from the body. They are used in sports where the athletes are categorized by their body weight....."[33] Sports that have weight classes include wrestling, boxing, judo, and weightlifting. Diuretics also aid in diluting an athlete's urine "so that the presence of performance-enhancing drugs, or their metabolic counterparts, cannot be detected."[34]

Doping control — "The process including test distribution planning, *Sample* collection and handling, laboratory analysis, results management, hearings and appeals."[35] ("Doping control" is a term specific to WADA and the international sports community to describe efforts to eliminate the use of prohibited performanceenhancing substances and methods from sport.)[36]

Enhancement of oxygen transfer — An athlete may increase his body's oxygen capacity either by "artificially enhancing the uptake, transport, or delivery of oxygen," such as through the ingestion of erythorpoietin (see below), or through blood doping.[37] Blood doping involves the administration of blood cells. "Two to four units (one unit corresponds to 450 ml [milliliters] of whole blood are collected from the individual ... [and then] three to five days before the competition [the blood is] infused [into the individual]."[38]

Ephedra — "Ephedra is a plant that contains the chemical ephedrine, a stimulant similar to amphetamines. Athletes may take an over-the-counter supplement containing ephedra to reduce physical fatigue, lose weight or improve mental alertness."[39]

Epitestosterone — Epitestosterone, which is a natural steroid, plays an important role in testing an individual for the presence of excess testosterone. The ratio of testosterone to epitestosterone (T/E) usually is 1:1. A ratio of 6:1 or higher generally is an indication of illegal supplementation of testosterone.[40] (However, the World Anti-Doping Agency lowered its T/E threshold to 4:1 in 2005.[41])

Erythropoietin (EPO) — EPO, which is an alternative to blood doping, stimulates red blood cell production. It increases an individual's aerobic power by increasing the number of his or her red blood cells to "unnatural levels."[42]

Gene doping — "The non-therapeutic use of genes, genetic elements or of the modulation of gene expression, having the capacity to enhance athletic performance ....[43] This includes attempts to modulate hormonal control of production of normal substances in the body, such as growth hormone or erythropoietin."[44]

Glucocorticosteroids — "Glucocorticosteroids are powerful anti-inflammatory agents, [45] [which] affect the metabolism, and athletes may use them to get more energy."[46] Glucocorticosteroids are also known as glucocorticoids.

Human chorionic gonadotropin (hCG) — In males, hCG helps to stimulate the production of male hormones such as testosterone.[47] Male athletes may take hCG "to increase the ability of their body to produce testosterone and to prevent atrophy of the testicles that results from taking large doses of anabolic steroids."[48]

Human growth hormone (hGH) — HGH is "the hormone ... responsible for growth and when administered to an adult whose growth has stopped increases protein synthesis."[49] Athletes might use it to "induce anabolic effects, reduce muscle cell breakdown and reduce body fat."[50]

Insulin — Insulin is used by individuals who have diabetes to manage their blood sugar levels. Some athletes may use insulin in an effort "to increase muscle growth and improve muscle definition."[51]

Masking agents — "Substances that are used to prevent the detection of other substances or methods used by an athlete in doping. An example would be the attempt to change the pH of the urine to enhance excretion of a doping substance."[52]

Mimetics — Synthetic compounds "that produce the same (or a very similar effect) as another (especially a naturally occurring) compound."[53]

Pharmacological, chemical, and physical manipulation — "Pharmacological, chemical and physical manipulation is the *Use* of substances and methods, including masking agents, which alter, attempt to alter or may reasonably be expected to alter the integrity and validity of specimens collected in doping controls. These include but are not limited to catheterization, urine substitution and/or tampering, inhibition of renal excretion and alterations of testosterone and epitestosterone concentrations."[54] Manipulation may include "the addition of chemicals or other contaminants to the actual specimen following collection, with the intent of preventing the detection of a doping substance ...."[55] (This is an illustrative description. The actual substances and methods considered to constitute manipulation may vary from organization (or professional sports league) to organization.)

Precursor — "Steroid precursors are substances that are converted in the body into steroids ...."[56]

Prohormone — "A natural precursor of a hormone;[57] any substance that can be converted into a hormone."[58]

Steroids — "A class of compounds with common elements of their chemical structures, but wide ranging effects. *Androgenic-anabolic steroids* are the hormones responsible for secondary male sex characteristics; *estrogens* are the hormones responsible for development and maintenance of female secondary sex characteristics; *glucocorticosteroids* regulate carbohydrate, fat and protein metabolism; *mineralocorticoids* regulate the balance of water and electrolytes. In addition, steroids have been used for a variety of medical purposes, including reducing inflammation."[59] Also see "anabolic androgenic steroids."

Stimulants — "Stimulants are substances that act directly on the central nervous system to speed up parts of the brain and body."[60] Stimulants "can reduce fatigue, suppress appetite, and increase alertness and aggressiveness."[61]

Testosterone — "Testosterone is the main male hormone that maintains muscle mass and strength ...."[62]

REFERENCES

[1] Charles E. Yesalis, William A. Anderson, William E. Buckley, and James E. Wright, *Incidence of the Nonmedical Use of Anabolic-Androgenic Steroids*, research monograph 102, U.S. Dept. of Health and Human Services, National Institute on Drug Abuse (Washington: GPO, 1990), pp. 97-98; Charles E. Yesalis and Michael S. Bahrke, "History of Doping in Sport," in *Performance-Enhancing Substances in Sport and Exercise*, Michael S. Bahrke and Charles E. Yesalis, eds. (Champaign, IL: Human Kinetics, 2002), pp. 1-2.

[2] Yesalis and Bahrke, "History of Doping in Sport," p. 1. (Italics in original.)

[3] World Anti-Doping Agency, "A Brief History of Anti-Doping," n.d., available online at [http://www.wada-ama.org/en/dynamic.ch2?page Category_id=20].

[4] Ibid., p. 2.

[5] U.S. Congress, House Committee on Government Reform, statement of Paul Tagliabue, Commissioner, National Football League, and Harold Henderson, Executive Vice President — Labor Relations,

National Football League, unpublished hearing, 109th Cong., 1st. sess., Apr. 28, 2005, p. 5.

[6] Information provided by the NBA's Basketball Communications Office to the author on May 19, 2004.

[7] Efforts to obtain a copy of the National Hockey League's program, *NHL/NHLPA* [National Hockey League Players Association] *Substance Abuse and Behavioral Health Program* (SABHP) were unsuccessful. It is unclear whether this program includes performanceenhancing substances. This program took effect in September 1996 and apparently expired on September 15, 2004, when the collective bargaining agreement negotiated by the NHL and the players association expired.

[8] In 1999, the International Olympic Committee (IOC) convened a World Conference on Doping in Sport, which produced the Lausanne Declaration on Doping in Sport. The World Anti-Doping Agency (WADA) was established, pursuant to the Lausanne Declaration, on Nov. 10, 1999. (World Anti-Doping Agency, "WADA History," n.d., available at [http://www.wada-ama.org/en/dynamic.ch2?pageCategory _id=12].) The U.S. Anti-Doping Agency (USADA), which began operations Oct. 1, 2000, was created as a result of recommendations made by the U.S. Olympic Committee's Select Task Force on Externalization. It is responsible for anti-doping efforts within the U.S. Olympic movement. Specifically, USADA has the authority to test and educate U.S. Olympic, Paralympic, and Pan American athletes, adjudicate appeals, and conduct research in support of its antidoping efforts. (U.S. Anti-Doping Agency, "USADA History," n.d., available at [http://www.usantidoping.org/who/history.html]; U.S. Anti-Doping Agency, "USADA Mission," available at [http://www.usanti doping.org/who/mission.html].) The Paralympics "are a multi-sport, multi-disability competition of elite, world-class, disabled athletes. Although similar in scope to the Olympic Games, the Paralympic Games provide an elite competition opportunity to athletes with a functional disability, which precludes their involvement in open competition of the Olympic Games." (U.S. Olympic Committee, "Paralympic Overview," n.d., available at [http://www.usoc.org/ education/paralympic_overview/paralympicindex.htm].) The Pan American Sports Organization (PAS) consists of 42 nations of Central, North, and South America, and the Caribbean. "The Pan American Games are held every four years just like the Olympic Games and precede the Games by a year. The Pan American Games consist of all

summer Olympic sports, plus some non-Olympic sports, and serve as an Olympic-qualifying event for many of the participating sports." (U.S. Olympic Committee, "Pan American Games Overview," n.d., available at [http://www.olympic-usa.org/education/ panamoverview/ panindex.htm].)

[9] For example, the Olympic prohibition against beta-blockers applies to 18 sports (and only during competitions) including archery, curling, and gymnastics. (World Anti-Doping Agency, *The 2005 Prohibited List, International Standard*, n.d., available online at [http://www.wada-ama.org/rtecontent/document/list_book_2005_en.pdf], p. 18.)

[10] An athlete who has been banned under the WADA *Code* has been declared ineligible. An athlete's status during eligibility is as follows: "No Person who has been declared ineligible may, during the period of ineligibility, participate in any capacity in a Competition or activity (other than authorized anti-doping education or rehabilitation programs) authorized or organized by a Signatory or Signatory's member organization" (p. 35). Signatories are those organizations that have signed and agreed to comply with the WADA *Code* and include "the International Olympic Committee, International Federations, International Paralympic Committee, National Olympic Committees, National Paralympic Committees, Major Event Organizations, National Anti-Doping Organizations, and WADA." (World Anti-Doping Agency, *World Anti-Doping Code*, pp. 35, 75.) For example, the list of organizations that have accepted the WADA *Code* includes the International Fencing Federation, International Swimming Federation, International Tennis Federation, and the International Wrestling Federation. (World Anti-Doping Agency, "List of Sports Organizations Who Have Accepted the Code," n.d., available at [http://www.wadaama. org/en/print.asp?p=42255].)

[11] The federal government has established five schedules of controlled substances. The following three criteria are used to determine on which schedule to place a substance or drug: its potential for abuse, whether the item has a currently accepted medical use in the United States, and the probability that abuse of the substance could lead to physical or psychological dependence. Schedule I includes substances and drugs that have a high potential for abuse, that currently have no accepted medical use in the United States, and that lack accepted safety for use under medical supervision. Substances and drugs listed on one of the remaining four schedules have currently accepted

medical uses, and the potential for abuse and the probability that abuse could lead to physical or psychological dependence declines from Schedule II through Schedule IV. (21 U.S.C. § 812(a) and (b).)

[12] R. Craig Kammerer, "Drug Testing in Sport and Exercise," in *Performance-Enhancing Substances in Sport and Exercise*, p. 330.

[13] In early summer 2003, USADA received a syringe from an individual who claimed to be a track and field coach. The then-anonymous coach also provided the names of American and international athletes that he alleged had used an undetectable steroid. USADA forwarded the contents of the syringe to the UCLA Olympic Analytic Laboratory, a WADA accredited laboratory, for analysis. Dr. Don Catlin, head of the laboratory, determined that the substance was a designer steroid, meaning that it could not be detected by normal laboratory testing. The UCLA laboratory determined that the substance was tetrahydrogestrinone (THG) and developed a test for THG. (U.S. Anti-Doping Agency, "U.S. Anti-Doping Statement on Doping Case with Designer Steroids," press release, Oct. 16, 2003, available at [http://www.usantidoping.org/files/active/resources/press_releases/ PressRelease_10_16_2003.pdf].) USADA has alleged that the source of THG was the Area Laboratory Co-Operative (BALCO), which is located in Burlingame, CA. Internal Revenue Service agents raided BALCO in September 2003. (Mark Asher, "Bonds to Testify on Supplement Supplier," *Washington Post*, Oct. 22, 2003, p. D2.) As reported by the *Washington Post*, the Department of Justice initiated an investigation of BALCO in 2003, and the Senate Committee on Commerce requested and received information from the department's investigation. (Amy Shipley, "Olympic Officials to Request Federal Files," *Washington Post*, May 5, 2004, p. D9; Amy Shipley, "USADA Bans White for 2 Years," *Washington Post*, May 202, 2004, p. D5.)

[14] Maske and Shapiro, "NFL Strengthens Steroid Policy," p. D8.

[15] Major League Baseball, *Major League Baseball's Joint Drug Prevention and Treatment Program*, n.d., pp. 3 and 6, available at [http://reform.house.gov/UploadedFiles/ 031705%20MLB%20Policy .pdf]. See **Table 1** for additional information. Major League Baseball's policy states: "In the event that any HPAC [Health Policy Advisory Committee] member has information that gives him/her reasonable cause to believe that a Player has, in the previous 12-month period, engaged in the use, possession, sale or distribution of a Prohibited Substance, such member shall immediately request a meeting (or conference call) to present such information to the other

HPAC members. If HPAC agress bya majority vote that such reasonable cause exists, the Player will be subejct to immediate testing ...." (Major League Baseball, *Major League Baseball's Joint Drug Prevention and Treatment Program*, n.d., p. 6, available at [http://reform.house.gov/UploadedFiles/031705%20MLB%20Policy.pdf].)

[16] Major League Baseball, *Major League Baseball's Joint Drug Prevention and Treatment Program*, n.d., pp. 11-12.

[17] R. Craig Kammerer, "Drug Testing in Sport and Exercise," in *Performance-Enhancing Substances in Sport and Exercise*, pp. 330-331. As noted below (**Table 1**, footnote g.), a blood-based test for human growth hormone has been developed.

[18] World Anti-Doping Agency, *World Anti-Doping Code*, 2003, available online at [http://www.wada-ama.org/rtecontent/document/code_v3.pdf], p. 1.

[19] Ibid., p. 3.

[20] National Football League, *National Football League Policy on Anabolic Steroids and Related Substances*, 2003 (as amended May 15, 2003), p. 1.

[21] U.S. Congress, Senate Committee on Commerce, Science and Transportation, *Steroid Use in Professional and Amateur Sports*, Mar. 10, 2004, 108th Cong., 2nd sess., statement of Terry Madden, Chief Executive Officer, United States Anti-Doping Agency, unpublished, available at [http://commerce.senate.gov/hearings/witnesslist.cfm?id=1100].

[22] U.S. Congress, Senate Committee on Commerce, Science, and Transportation, *Effects of Performance Enhancing Drugs on the Health of Athletes and Athletic Competition*, 106th Cong., 1st sess., Oct. 20, 1999 (Washington: GPO, 2002), p. 21.

[23] Steve Fawner, "A Search for Truth in Substance," *Washington Post*, Dec. 4, 2003, pp. D1, D10.

[24] U.S. Anti-Doping Agency, *2005 Guide to Prohibited Substances and Prohibited Methods of Doping*, p. 25; William N. Taylor, *Anabolic Steroids and the Athlete*, 2nd ed. (Jefferson, NC: McFarland and Co., 2002), p. 35.

[25] Michael S. Bahrke and Charles E. Yesalis, "Anabolics," in *Performance-Enhancing Substances in Sport and Exercise*, p. 33.

[26] National Institutes of Health, National Institute on Drug Abuse, "NIDA InfoFacts: Steroids (Anabolic-Androgenic)," n.d., available at [http://www.nida.nih.gov/Infofax/steroids.html].

[27] U.S. Anti-Doping Agency, "Medical," n.d., available at [http://www.usantidoping.org/resources/glossary/medical.aspx].
[28] Australian Sports Drug Agency, "Fact Sheet: Hormones and Related Substances," n.d., available at [http://www.asda.org.au/athletes/sub_fact_sheets/hormones.htm].
[29] U.S. Anti-Doping Agency, "Medical."
[30] Australian Sports Drug Agency, "Fact Sheet: Beta-2 Agonists," n.d., available at [http://www.asda.org.au/athletes/sub_fact_sheets/beta2.htm]; Gordon S. Lynch, "Beta-2 Agonists," in *Performance-Enhancing Substances in Sport and Exercise*, p. 47.
[31] U.S. Anti-Doping Agency, "Medical."
[32] Australian Sports Drug Agency, "Fact Sheet: Beta Blockers," n.d., available at [http://www.asda.org.au/athletes/sub_fact_sheets/beta.htm].
[33] U.S. Anti-Doping Agency, "Medical."
[34] Lawrence E. Armstrong, "Diuretics," in *Performance-Enhancing Substances in Sport and Exercise*, p. 111.
[35] World Anti-Doping Agency, *International Standard for Testing*, p. 8.
[36] Information provided electronically by the U.S. Anti-Doping Agency to the author on Apr. 8, 2005.
[37] U.S. Anti-Doping Agency, *2005 Guide to Prohibited Substances and Prohibited Methods of Doping*, 2004, p. 10, available at [http://www.usantidoping.org/athletes/downloads.aspx?cid=2].
[38] Björn T. Ekblom, "Blood Doping," in *Performance-Enhancing Substances in Sport and Exercise*, pp. 94-95; U.S. Anti-Doping Agency, "Medical."
[39] Mayo Clinic, "Teen Athletes and Performance-Enhancing Substances: What Parents Can Do," Dec. 22, 2004, available at [http://www.mayoclinic.com/involke.cfm?id=SM00045].
[40] R. Craig Kammerer, "Drug Testing in Sport and Exercise," in *Performance-Enhancing Substances in Sport and Exercise*, p. 328.
[41] World Anti-Doping Agency, *The 2005 Prohibited List International Standard*, n.d., p. 7, available at [http://www.wada-ama.org/en/dynamic.ch2?pageCategory_id=174].
[42] National Center on Addiction and Substance Abuse at Columbia University, *Winning at Any Cost: Doping in Olympic Sports*, Sept. 2000 (New York: Columbia University), pp. 24-25; U.S. Anti-Doping Agency, *2005 Guide to Prohibited Substances and Prohibited Methods of Doping*, p. 49.

[43] U.S. Anti-Doping Agency, *2005 Guide to Prohibited Substances and Prohibited Methods of Doping*, p. 10.
[44] Ibid., p. 29.
[45] Australian Sports Drug Agency, "Fact Sheet: Glucocorticosteroids," n.d., avaialble at [http://www.asda.org.au/athletes/sub_fact_sheets/glucocorticosteroids.htm].
[46] Information provided electronically by the U.S. Anti-Doping Agency to the author on Apr. 1, 2005.
[47] U.S. National Library of Medicine and National Institutes of Health, Medline Plus, "Drug Information: Chorionic Gonadotropin (Systemic)," Jan. 21, 2004, available at [http://www.nlm.nih.gov/medlineplus/druginfo/uspdi/202266.html].
[48] Cynthia Kuhn, Scott Swartzwelder, and Wilkie Wilson, *Pumped* (New York: W.W. Norton and Co., 2000), p. 83.
[49] U.S. Anti-Doping Agency, *2005 Guide to Prohibited Substances and Prohibited Methods of Doping*, p. 49.
[50] Australian Sports Drug Agency, "Fact Sheet: Human Growth Hormone (hGH)," n.d., available at [http://www.asda.org.au/athletes/sub_fact_sheets/human.htm].
[51] Australian Sports Drug Agency, "Fact Sheet: Insulin," available at [http://www. asda.org.au/athletes/sub_fact_sheets/insulin.htm].
[52] U.S. Anti-Doping Agency, *2005 Guide to Prohibited Substances and Prohibited Methods of Doping*, p. 26.
[53] *Oxford English Dictionary Online*, available at [http://dictionary.oed.com].
[54] U.S. Anti-Doping Agency, *2004 United States Anti-Doping Agency Guide to Prohibited Substances and Prohibited Methods of Doping*, 2003, p. 19. (Italics in original.)
[55] U.S. Anti-Doping Agency, *2005 Guide to Prohibited Substances and Prohibited Methods of Doping*, 2004, p. 26.
[56] U.S. Olympic Committee, "USA Luge Joins Coalition Formed to Support Dietary Supplement Regulation," press release, Apr. 24, 2003, available online at [http://www.usolympicteam.com/73_8410.htm].
[57] *Oxford English Dictionary Online*, available at [http://dictionary.oed.com].
[58] *Dorland's Illustrated Medical Dictionary*.
[59] Information provided electronically by the U.S. Anti-Doping Agency to the author on Apr. 8, 2005. (Italics in original.)

[60] Australian Sports Drug Agency, "Fact Sheet: Stimulants," n.d., available at [http://www.asda.org.au/athletes/sub_fact_sheets/stimulants.htm].

[61] Mayo Clinic, "Performance-Enhancing Drugs: Dangerous, Damaging and Potentially Deadly."

[62] Mayo Clinic, "Testosterone Therapy: The Answer for Aging Men?" Apr. 13, 2004, available at [http://www.mayoclinic.com/invoke.cfm?id=MC00030].

Chapter 2

FEDERALLY MANDATED RANDOM DRUG TESTING IN PROFESSIONAL ATHLETICS: CONSTITUTIONAL ISSUES[*]

Charles V. Dale
Legislative Attorney American Law Division

SUMMARY

Problems of usage of steroids and other performance enhancing drugs in professional and amateur athletics have been the focus of a series of investigative hearings before the House Government Reform Committee. The Committee began taking evidence on March 17, 2005, when several former and current players, medical experts, and major league baseball executives were summoned to testify in the first hearing. Committee Chairman Tom Davis has urged all sports leagues to "acknowledge that their testing programs need improvement" and has framed bipartisan legislation to establish a uniform testing policy for major professional sports leagues. Currently, there are four professional athletic drug testing bills before Congress: S. 1114 (Senator McCain); H.R. 2565 (Representative Davis); H.R. 1862 (Representative Stearns); and H.R. 2516 (Representative Sweeney). The McCain and Davis bills

---

[*] Excerpted from CRS Report RL32911, dated June 27, 2005.

are virtually identical, and all four bills would establish minimum drug standards – including random testing – for some professional sports leagues.

Congressionally mandated drug-testing requirements for both public employees and workers in private industry subject to federal regulation have a fairly long and well established legal history. Nonetheless, the federal courts have recognized limits, largely anchored in constitutional privacy interests of affected workers, that circumscribe governmental authority to impose suspicionless random testing requirements in the public or private sectors. These decisions establish that "compelling" governmental interests may, in appropriate circumstances, override constitutional objections to testing procedures by employees whose privacy expectations are diminished by the nature of their duties or workplace scrutiny to which they are otherwise subject. They further suggest, however, that substantial constitutional difficulties probably confront any broad-based testing program that is not limited to specific occupational categories or to persons for whom the government is able to demonstrate some special need to test.

It could be argued that professional players have a diminished expectation of privacy as the consequence of league or association rules that already require routine physical examinations and testing for drugs in certain circumstances. Moreover, a separate argument could be made that safety and health concerns associated with steroid usage, and the importance of professional athletes as role models for the nation's youth, justify unannounced testing for anabolic steroids or other controlled substances. Testing of randomly selected athletes may also be the least intrusive route to an effective steroid detection program. Past major league baseball procedures, it has been argued, do not deter steroid use. Moreover, arguably, the reasonable suspicion standard may be unworkable since most often there may be no outward symptoms to signal the use of steroids.

Problems of usage of steroids and other performance enhancing drugs in professional and amateur athletics have been the focus of a series of investigative hearings before the House Government Reform Committee. The Committee began taking evidence on March 17, 2005, when several former and current players, medical experts, and major league baseball executives were summoned to testify in the first hearing. National Football League Commissioner Paul Tagliabue next testified, on April 27th, concerning details of the NFL steroid testing procedures and how they were negotiated between the league and the NFL players' union. The Committee also requested summaries of all test results during the period that testing has been in place, although not the names of individual players. Similar requests have reportedly been made of National Basketball Association, National Hockey League, US Soccer Federation, Major League Soccer, Association of Tennis Professionals, USA Track and Field, and USA Cycling. Committee Chairman Tom Davis has urged all sports leagues to "acknowledge that their testing programs need improvement" and has framed bi-partisan legislation to establish a uniform testing policy for major professional sports leagues.[1] Currently, there are four professional athletic drug testing bills before Congress: S. 1114 (Senator McCain); H.R. 2565 (Representative Davis); H.R. 1862 (Representative Stearns); and H.R. 2516 (Representative Sweeney). The McCain and Davis bills are virtually identical, and all four bills would establish minimum drug standards – including random testing – for some professional sports leagues.

The McCain/Davis proposal, for example, would require "major professional sports leagues" – defined to include Major League Baseball, the National Football League, the National Basketball Association, and the National Hockey League, and any "successor leagues" – to implement independently administered drug testing programs mirroring the standard of the United States Anti-Doping Agency (USADA). At a minimum, each professional athlete would have to be tested without advance notice no less than five times each calendar year, including at least two offseason tests. Each test would have to cover all substances prohibited in USADA's anti-doping code and would have to be analyzed at a USADA-approved lab.

Athletes testing positive (or refusing to test) a first time must be suspended a minimum of two years and would be subject to permanent suspension from the professional sports association for any later infraction. The leagues would be required to disclose positive tests and resulting penalties to the public. Each covered league would have to develop an adjudication process to provide the athlete who tests positive a hearing (after notice), representation of counsel, and the right to appeal. While such proceedings are pending, the athlete in question would be suspended. For a detailed discussion of all measures currently before Congress on the subject, see CRS Report RS22156, *Drug Testing in Sports: Proposed Legislation*, by Nathan Brooks.

Congressionally mandated drug testing requirements for both public employees and workers in private industry subject to federal regulation have a fairly long and well-established legal history. Nonetheless, as described more fully below, the federal courts have recognized limits, largely anchored in constitutional privacy interests of affected workers, that circumscribe governmental authority to impose suspicionless random testing requirements in the public or private sectors. This report examines relevant judicial precedents for their applicability to the issue of random testing for performance-enhancing substances in professional athletics.

CONSTITUTIONAL BACKGROUND

Constitutional law on the subject of governmentally mandated drug-testing is primarily an outgrowth of the Fourth Amendment prohibition on unreasonable searches and seizures.[2] A judicial exception to traditional requirements of a warrant and individualized suspicion for "administrative" searches has been applied to random drug testing of government employees, and of private employees tested pursuant to government regulation. In the employment setting, such testing has been justified under a "special needs" analysis, which the courts have applied in relatively narrow circumstances directly implicating "compelling" public safety, law enforcement, or national security interests of the government. More generalized governmental concerns for the "integrity" or efficient operation of the public workplace have usually not been deemed sufficient to justify interference with the "reasonable expectation of privacy" of workers or other individuals to be tested.

The Supreme Court in 1989 applied the "special needs" doctrine to dispense with the normal warrant and probable cause requirements of the Fourth Amendment when the government demonstrates compelling justification "beyond ordinary law enforcement" for an employee drug testing program. In *National Treasury Employees Union v. Von Raab*,[3] extraordinary safety and national security concerns justified urinalysis testing of Customs Service employees seeking transfer or promotion to positions directly linked to drug interdiction, handling classified information, or the carriage of firearms. Similarly, in *Skinner v. Railway Labor Executives' Ass'n*,[4] neither a warrant nor particularized suspicion was required for a Federal Railway Administration (FRA) program of blood and urine tests for railroad employees involved in accidents or who violated certain safety standards. In both cases, the Court emphasized that special needs analysis applied only where testing was not used as a prosecutorial tool. In *Veronia School District v. Acton*,[5] the Supreme Court first approved of random drug testing procedures – for high school student athletes rather than public employees – a holding that it later extended to permit random drug testing of students participating in non-athletic extracurricular activities as well. However, the Court distinguished earlier rulings when, in *Chandler v. Miller*,[6] it voided a Georgia law requiring drug testing of candidates for state office because no "special need" substantial enough to warrant suspicionless searches was shown.

The Supreme Court in *Skinner* discarded the reasonable suspicion standard for testing within industries that are "pervasively regulated." The rationale is that the existence of extensive federal or state regulation in and of itself diminishes the reasonable expectation of privacy of those involved in the industry. The primary issue before the lower courts in *Shoemaker v. Handel*[7] was whether state-mandated drug and alcohol tests, administered without individualized suspicion, to thoroughbred race horse jockeys by the New Jersey Racing Commission, violated the Fourth Amendment.

The district court upheld the program, finding that the jockeys voluntarily participated in horse racing and that the state had shown a compelling need for conducting the tests. First, the court recognized that horse racing was a unique class of industry subject to "heavy" state regulation. Second, jockeys were licensed by the state and had received notice of the implementation of the tests. Although notice and licensure did not serve as a waiver of Fourth Amendment rights, they were factors to be considered in balancing the jockey's expectations of privacy against the needs of the state. Third, the state had a vital interest in ensuring that the horse racing industry was run honestly and safely and that the public perceived it as such. Finally, the jockeys tested were selected by random drawing not subject to the bias or discretion of test administrators.

The Third Circuit Court of Appeals affirmed the district court decision. In particular, the appellate opinion emphasized the pervasiveness of New Jersey state regulation and the state's "strong" interest in preserving the "integrity" of the horse-racing industry. In assessing the reasonableness of the testing scheme, the *Shoemaker* court found that the integrity of a sport, from which large sums of revenue were collected, outweighed the jockeys' individual privacy interests.

> New Jersey has a strong interest in assuring the public of the integrity of persons engaged in the horse racing industry. Public confidence forms the foundation for the success of an industry based on wagering. Frequent alcohol and drug testing is an effective means of demonstrating that persons in the horse racing industry are not subject to certain outside influences. It is the public's perception, not the known suspicion, that triggers the state's strong interest in conducting warrantless testing.[8]

Summing up, the Third Circuit concluded that to justify governmentally imposed random testing, there must be a "strong state interest" in the search and "the pervasive regulation of the industry must have reduced the justifiable privacy expectation of the subject of the search."[9] Other post-*Shoemaker* rulings are in agreement.[10]

In *Veronia School District v. Acton*, [11] the Supreme Court sustained a random drug-testing program for high school students engaged in interscholastic athletic competition. The Student Athlete Drug Policy required mandatory and random suspicionless urinalysis testing of all student athletes within the district. The purpose of the policy was to protect the health and safety of the athletes and to rehabilitate drug users by enrolling them in a drug assistance program. All students wanting to participate in a school-sponsored sports team had to provide a consent form, signed both by the student and his or her parents, acquiescing in the tests. Each athlete was tested at the beginning of the athletic season, and anytime during the season that such student's name was randomly selected. Ten percent of the athletes were randomly drawn each week from a pool for testing.

The Supreme Court found that the privacy interest of high school student athletes is diminished by "an element of 'communal undress' inherent in athletic competition." "School sports are not for the bashful," and by choosing to participate in athletics the students "voluntarily subject themselves to a degree of regulation even higher than that imposed on students generally."[12] Moreover, an "immediate crisis," caused by "a sharp increase in drug use" in the school district, triggered installation of the program. District Court findings established that student athletes were not only "among the drug users," they were "leaders of the drug culture."[13] The opinion emphasized that "students within the school environment have a lesser expectation of privacy than members of the public generally."[14]

Balanced against this diminished expectation, the Court determined that the state's interest in protecting the physical and mental well-being of student athletes while in state custody was "important – indeed perhaps compelling." In this regard, the program's context was "central" to Justice Scalia's majority opinion. Local government bears large "responsibilities, under a public school system, as guardian and tutor of children entrusted to its care."[15] Because of this "custodial and tutelary" relationship between the government and its students, school officials regularly exercise "a degree of supervisory control that could not be exercised over free adults."

In *Board of Education v. Earls*,[16] the Court pressed the *Veronia School District* rationale one step further, finding that because of its unique relationship with students, the state's interest in preventing drug use outweighs the privacy interest of students participating in any competitive extracurricular activities. In addition, *Earls* noted "this Court has not required a particularized or pervasive drug problem before allowing the government to conduct suspicionless drug testing"[17] and would not set a threshold level of drug abuse sufficient to support a drug testing program. Instead, the Court found that prevention of harm to school children tested sufficed to demonstrate the necessity for a drug testing policy.

PERFORMANCE ENHANCING DRUGS IN PROFESSIONAL SPORTS

These decisions establish that "compelling" governmental interests may, in appropriate circumstances, override constitutional objections to testing procedures by employees whose privacy expectations are diminished by the nature of their duties or workplace scrutiny to which they are otherwise subject. They further suggest, however, that substantial constitutional difficulties probably confront any broadbased testing program that is not limited to specific occupational categories or to persons for whom the government is able to demonstrate some special need to test. A special need has generally been found where there is a history of drug abuse in an industry, when the employment involves work in safety-sensitive or high risk positions, or where there is evidence that drug use has led to accidents or other dangers to the public welfare. But, as Justice Scalia suggests in *Veronia School District,* the concept may be sufficiently elastic to encompass any "interest that appears *important enough* to justify the particular search at hand, in light of other factors that show the search to be relatively intrusive upon a genuine expectation of privacy."[18] As such, the legality of any mandatory testing regime may depend upon the range of governmental interests that the Court ultimately declares to be "compelling" for Fourth Amendment purposes, and how close the required "nexus" to such interests must be to justify random testing of specific individuals or groups.

The application of the *Shoemaker* precedent would seem to require judicial recognition that professional sports, like horse racing involved there, is a "closely regulated industry." While professional baseball, football, and hockey may be subject to union collective bargaining agreements and other largely self-imposed owners' association and league rules, the hand of government in day- to-day team governance and control appears to be far less. Instead, owners individually and in association remain largely free to set their own standards for player conduct and team management, and even enjoy some limited exemptions from federal regulation – antitrust, for example – that apply to other business sectors. Nor, unlike the jockeys in *Shoemaker*, are professional baseball or football players licensed by state or federal authorities, a potentially relevant distinction. In short, the position of the professional athlete may be readily distinguishable from the jockeys in *Shoemaker* and railroad workers in *Skinner*. For similar reasons, the "custodial and tutelary" relationship of the state to student athletes would appear to deprive *Veronia School District* and its progeny of direct precedential (though perhaps not persuasive) value.

Even apart from governmental regulation, however, it could be countered that professional players have a diminished expectation of privacy as the consequence of league or association rules that already require routine physical examinations and testing for drugs in certain circumstances. Moreover, a separate argument could be made that safety and health concerns associated with steroid usage, and the importance of professional athletes as role models for the nation's youth, justify unannounced testing for anabolic steroids or other controlled substances. Medical evidence could be mustered in the course of ongoing congressional hearings of the adverse health effects, not only to the steroid users, but to the safety of other players. Second, it could be argued, protecting the integrity of the game may be particularly important given the demonstrable influence of professional athletes on young players at all levels. The NFL, for example, cites three reasons, including the health of players, for its concern about the use of prohibited substances.

> [They] threaten the fairness and integrity of the athletic competition on the playing field . . . [T]he League is concerned with the adverse health effects of steroid use. Although research is continuing, steroid use has been linked to a number of physiological, psychological, orthopedic, reproductive, and other serious health problems . . . [T]he use of Prohibited Substances by NFL players sends the wrong message to young people who may be tempted to use them.[19]

Thus, both the NFL and World Anti-Doping Agency have acknowledged that steroid use can undermine the health of athletes and the fairness of athletic competition.

Finally, testing of randomly selected athletes may be the least intrusive route to an effective steroid detection program. "It seems to us self-evident that a drug problem largely fueled by the 'role model' effect of athletes' drug use, and of particular danger to athletes, is effectively addressed by making sure that athletes do not use drugs."[20] Past major league baseball procedures, it appears, do not deter steroid use. Moreover, arguably, the reasonable suspicion standard may be unworkable since most often there may be no outward symptoms to signal the use of steroids. Thus, the suspicionless, administrative search exception might be the only means of effectively deterring athletes from using steroids. In addition, it may avoid possible problems of subjectivity and prejudice that arguably attend the application of "reasonable cause" or other suspicionbased standards.

REFERENCES

[1] 4/28/05 Phila. Daily News 70, 2005 WLNR 6611442.
[2] Drug testing programs have also been challenged under the First, Fifth, and Fourteenth Amendments, based on arguments that the testing procedures or some other aspect of the program violated rights to due process, equal protection, privacy, and freedom of religion. In general, such claims have proven unsuccessful where the testing program included legal safeguards, such as the use of non-discriminatory testing practices, chain of custody procedures, confidentiality, adequate notice, properly certified laboratories, confirmatory tests, and other procedures designed to ensure fairness and to minimize the intrusiveness of the drug testing program. See, e.g. Shoemaker v. Handel, 795 F.2d 1136, 1139-41, 1143 (referring to selective enforcement of urine testing of jockeys as denying them equal protection of the laws); Rushton v. Nebraska Pub. Power District, 844 F.2d 562, 564-66 (8th Cir. 1988)(discussing plaintiffs' contention that the drug testing program violated their First Amendment rights).
[3] 489 U.S. 656 (1989).
[4] 489 U.S. 602 (1989).
[5] 515 U.S. 646 (1995).
[6] 520 U.S. 305 (1997).
[7] 619 F. Supp. 1089 (D.N.J. 1985), aff'd, 795 F.2d 1136 (3d Cir. 1986).
[8] Id. at 1142.
[9] Id.
[10] See e.g. Dimeo v. Griffin, 943 F.2d 679 (7th Cir 1991)(en banc) where the full appeals court upheld a similar rule of the Illinois Racing Board on behalf of jockeys and other horse racing participants required to

submit to suspicionless drug testing. In striking a balance between the intrusiveness of the rule and the Board's reasons for it, the court cited the state's substantial interest in promoting the safety of participants as well as protecting financial revenue which it derive from the betting public's interest in a "clean" sport. The opinion also stressed that since jockeys and other participants were subject to frequent medical examinations, they had a diminished expectation of privacy, which was outweighed by the state's interests in this case.

[11] 515 U.S. 646 (1995).
[12] Id. at 650.
[13] Id at 649.
[14] Id. at 657.
[15] Id. at 665.
[16] 536 U.S. 822 (2002)
[17] Id. at 835.
[18] Id. at 661 (emphasis in original).
[19] National Football League, National Football League Policy on Anabolic Steroids and Related Substances, 2003 (as amended May 15, 2003), p. 1. Similarly, one of the purposes of the World Anti-Doping Program and the World Anti-Doping Code is "[t]o protect the Athletes' fundamental right to participate in doping-free sport and thus promote health, fairness, and equality for Athletes worldwide. . ." World Anti-Doping Agency, World Anti- Doping Code, 2003, available online at [http://www.wadaama.org/rtecontent/document/code_v3.pdf], p. 1.
[20] Veronia, 515 U.S. at 636.

In: Doping in Sports
Editor: C. N. Burns, pp. 47-53

ISBN 1-59454-683-5
© 2006 Nova Science Publishers, Inc.

Chapter 3

DRUG TESTING IN SPORTS: PROPOSED LEGISLATION[*]

Nathan Brooks
Legislative Attorney American Law Division

SUMMARY

Following a wave of allegations that the use of performance enhancing drugs by American athletes is growing, various congressional committees have held hearings on the effectiveness of the drug testing policies and procedures of professional sports leagues. Currently, there are four bills before Congress that would create mandatory minimum drug testing procedures for pro sports leagues: S. 1114; H.R. 2565; H.R. 1862; and H.R. 2516. This report provides a summary of these four bills.

INTRODUCTION

Following a wave of allegations that the use of performance enhancing drugs by American athletes is growing, various congressional committees

---

[*] Excerpted from CRS Report RS22156, dated June 10, 2005.

have held hearings on the effectiveness of the drug testing policies and procedures of professional sports leagues.[1] Currently, there are four bills before Congress: S. 1114 (Senator McCain); H.R. 2565 (Representative Davis); H.R. 1862 (Representative Stearns); and H.R. 2516 (Representative Sweeney). The McCain and Davis bills are virtually identical, and all four bills would establish minimum drug testing standards for some professional sports leagues. This report provides a summary of the four bills currently before Congress and a side-by-side comparison of their major provisions. It is noted at the outset that government-mandated random drug testing of pro athletes may raise some constitutional concerns.[2]

H.R. 2565. By statute, the authorization for the Office of National Drug Control Policy (ONDCP) expired in 2003,[3] although ONDCP has continued to operate through appropriation acts. The Davis bill would repeal the statutory sunset provision, so that ONDCP's authorization would be permanent.[4]

H.R. 2565 would require the "major professional sports leagues" – defined to include Major League Baseball, the National Football League, the National Basketball Association, and the National Hockey League, and any "successor leagues" – to implement independently administered drug testing programs mirroring the standard of the United States Anti-Doping Agency (USADA). Under the bill, the USADA standard would (at a minimum) have to provide for the testing of each professional athlete at least five times each calendar year. At least three of these tests would have to be administered in-season without advance notice, and at least two off-season without advance notice.[5] Each test would have to cover all substances prohibited in USADA's anti-doping code,[6] and each sample would have to be analyzed at a USADA-approved lab.[7]

A positive test would be any test in which a prohibited substance (or a metabolite or marker of a prohibited substance) is detected. In addition, if an athlete refuses to take a test or uses a method to obscure the testing results, then that would be considered a "positive test."[8] An athlete's first positive test would carry a two-year suspension with loss of pay, while a second positive test would result in a lifetime ban from all of the covered leagues.[9] The leagues would be required to disclose positive tests and resulting penalties to the public.[10]

Each covered league would be required to annually certify to the ONDCP Director that the league has consulted USADA in developing its adjudication process, which would have to provide the athlete who tests positive a hearing (after notice), representation of counsel, and the right to appeal. While such proceedings are pending, the athlete in question would be suspended.[11]

Each covered league would be required to annually certify to the ONDCP Director that the league has consulted with USADA in developing its testing distribution plan and drug testing protocols.[12]

The ONDCP Director would have the authority to modify the aforementioned standards, so long as the modifications would not reduce the effectiveness of the standards in curbing the abuse of performance-enhancing substances, or "diminish the leadership role of the United States" in eliminating such substances from sports.[13] Further, the Director could expand the number of leagues covered under the bill to include other pro sports leagues and NCAA Division I and II colleges and athletes.[14]

Under the Federal Trade Commission (FTC) Act,[15] the FTC has the authority to issue regulations proscribing certain activities as "unfair or deceptive acts or practices" affecting commerce.[16] The Davis bill would make a violation of the aforementioned testing standards an unfair or deceptive act under the FTC Act, and require the FTC to promulgate regulations to enforce the Clean Sports Act as if the FTC Act were incorporated into the Clean Sports Act.[17] The FTC would be empowered to levy fines of up to $1 million for failure to implement the required testing procedures.[18]

The Davis bill would require each covered league to report to Congress every two years on how the league's drug policy compares with that of USADA, number of players tested, etc. The ONDCP Director would be required to report to Congress from time to time on potential improvements to federal drug laws with respect to curbing the use of performance enhancing substances by athletes.[19] Further, both the Government Accountability Office (GAO) and the Commission on High School and College Athletics (which would be established by the ONDCP Director) would have to report to Congress on issues related to the use of performance enhancing substances by amateur athletes.[20]

S. 1114. S. 1114 is virtually identical to the Davis bill, except that it would not take the form of an amendment to the Office of National Drug Control Policy Act, nor would S. 1114 reauthorize the ONDCP.

H.R. 1862. The Stearns bill would include not only the four leagues covered in the McCain and Davis bills, but also Major League Soccer (MLS), the Arena Football League, "and any other league or association that organizes professional athletic competitions as the Secretary [of Commerce] may determine."[21]

H.R. 1862 would require the Secretary of Commerce to promulgate regulations governing testing for prohibited substances by covered leagues.[22] Under the bill, the regulations would have to require that every athlete be independently tested at least once a year – without notice – for substances prohibited by the World Anti-Doping Agency (WADA) and other substances determined by the Commerce Secretary to be performanceenhancing "for which testing is reasonable and practicable."[23]

The Stearns bill would require a two-year suspension without pay for the first positive test, and a lifetime ban from the individual league for the second positive test.[24] An athlete testing positive would have the right to appeal the result so long as he or she files such an appeal within five days of learning of the result. The league would then have 30 days in which to issue a decision. The aforementioned penalties would be stayed pending the appeals process.[25]

Covered leagues would have one year to adopt and enforce testing procedures that comply with the regulations issued by the Commerce Secretary. After this grace period ends, the Secretary could levy fines of up to $5 million for noncompliance, and add another $1 million for each additional day of noncompliance.[26]

The Commerce Secretary would be required to submit to Congress every two years a report on the effectiveness of the drug testing regulations. In addition, the Comptroller General would be required to conduct a study of the use of performance-enhancing substances by amateur athletes and submit to Congress a report on the study's findings and with recommendations as to extending the coverage of the Commerce Secretary's testing regulations to include amateur athletes.[27]

H.R. 2516. H.R. 2516 would make it illegal to organize *or participate in* a NBA, NFL, NHL, or MLB game without meeting the bill's testing requirements.[28] A violation would be treated as a violation of "a rule defining an unfair or deceptive trade act or practice" under the FTC Act, and the FTC would, accordingly, have the authority to enforce the bill's requirements. In addition, the FTC would have the authority to extend the bill's coverage to other pro sports leagues and the NCAA.[29]

The bill would require random testing of WADA-prohibited substances (including related metabolites and markers) and methods at least four times a year (twice in-season and twice out of season) and when the covered league has reason to suspect that an athlete or team is in violation of that league's drug policies. A refusal to submit to a drug test would be considered a positive test.[30]

A Side-by-Side Comparison of the Major Provisions of H.R. 2565, S. 1114, H.R. 1862, and H.R. 2516

	H.R. 2565	S. 1114	H.R. 1862	H.R. 2516
ONDCP Reauthorization?	Yes	No	No	No
Leagues Covered	MLB, NFL, NBA, NHL, and professional boxing	MLB, NFL, NBA, NHL, and professional boxing	MLB, NFL, NBA, NHL, MLS, Arena Football, and other leagues as determined by Secretary of Commerce	MLB, NFL, NBA, NHL
Benchmark Standard	USADA	USADA	WADA	WADA for Banned substances; USADA for testing and appeals procedures
Minimum Number of Tests Per Year	5	5	1	4
Maximum Fines for Failing to Implement Required Testing	$1 million	$1 million	$5 million, and another $1 million for each additional day not in compliance	No provision
Regulatory Oversight	ONDCP would be empowered to modify the bill's requirements, while FTC would have enforcement authority	ONDCP would be empowered to modify the bill's requirements, while FTC would have enforcement authority	Secretary of Commerce	FTC
Lab Analysis of Tests	USADA approved lab	USADA approved lab	No provision	WADA approved lab
Penalty for First Positive Test	Two year suspension without pay	Two year suspension without pay	Two year suspension without pay	Two year suspension without pay

A Side-by-Side Comparison (Continued)

	H.R. 2565	S. 1114	H.R. 1862	H.R. 2516
Penalty for Second Positive Test	Lifetime ban from all covered leagues	Lifetime ban from all covered leagues	Lifetime ban from the particular league in question	Lifetime ban from the particular league in question
Suspensions Stayed Pending Appeals?	No	No	Yes	No provision
Public Disclosure of Positive Tests?	Yes	Yes	No provision	Yes

REFERENCES

[1] For a comparison of some of the testing regimes used in professional and Olympic sports, see CRS Report RL32894, *Anti-Doping Policies: The Olympics and Selected Professional Sports*, by L. Elaine Halchin.

[2] See CRS Report RL32911, *Federally Mandated Random Drug Testing in Professional Athletics: Constitutional Issues*, by Charles V. Dale.

[3] 21 U.S.C. § 1712. See CRS Report RL32352, *War on Drugs: Reauthorization of the Office of National Drug Control Policy*, by Mark Eddy.

[4] H.R. 2565, § 102.

[5] H.R. 2565, § 201(a) (creating new § 724(b)(1) of P.L. 105-277). From the wording of the bill, it appears that tests beyond the minimum number could be administered with advance notice.

[6] Leagues would be allowed to make exceptions for properly prescribed substances. *Id.*

[7] H.R. 2565, § 201(a) (creating new § 724(b)(5) of P.L. 105-277).

[8] H.R. 2565, § 201(a) (creating new § 724(b)(6)(B) of P.L. 105-277).

[9] *Id.* The bill would allow for lesser penalties where an athlete unwittingly takes a prohibited substance, or where an athlete who tests positive helps the league track down those who are violating the drug policy or helping others to do so. *Id.*

[10] H.R. 2565, § 201(a) (creating new § 724(b)(9) of P.L. 105-277).

[11] H.R. 2565, § 201(a) (creating new § 724(b)(8) of P.L. 105-277).

[12] H.R. 2565, § 201(a) (creating new § 724(b)(2), (3) of P.L. 105-277).

[13] H.R. 2565, § 201(a) (creating new § 725 of P.L. 105-277).

[14]   *Id.* The Director could delegate the Director's duties under § 725 to another federal agency.
[15]   15 U.S.C. § 41 et seq.
[16]   *Id.* at § 57a.
[17]   H.R. 2656, § 201(a) (creating new § 726 of P.L. 105-277). The bill would also require the FTC to promulgate parallel regulations regarding professional boxing.
[18]   *Id.*
[19]   H.R. 2565, § 201(a) (creating new § 727 of P.L. 105-277).
[20]   H.R. 2565, § 201(a) (creating new §§ 729, 730 of P.L. 105-277).
[21]   H.R. 1862, § 2(2).
[22]   The Secretary would be empowered to exempt leagues that had previously implemented testing procedures that meet or exceed those listed in the Secretary's regulations. *Id.* at § 4.
[23]   *Id.* at §§ 3(1), (2).
[24]   *Id.* at § 3(4).
[25]   *Id.* at § 3(5).
[26]   *Id.* at § 5.
[27]   *Id.* at § 6.
[28]   H.R. 2516, § 4(a).
[29]   *Id.* at § 5.
[30]   *Id.* at § 4(b).
[31]   *Id.*
[32]   *Id.*
[33]   *Id.* at § 6.

Chapter 4

DIETARY SUPPLEMENTS: EPHEDRA[*]

Donna V. Porter
Specialist in Life Sciences Domestic Social Policy Division

SUMMARY

Ephedrine is a natural constituent of the herb ephedra and a synthetic compound present in certain over-the-counter drug products. The herbal form, known as Ma Huang in China, has been used as a remedy for asthma. In western cultures, ephedrine, the active drug product ingredient, has been used as a bronchodilator and decongestant for various respiratory problems. More recently, dietary supplements containing ephedra have been promoted for weight reduction and as a performance enhancer in body building and other sports.

Under the provisions of the Dietary Supplement Health and Education Act of 1994 (DSHEA), the Food and Drug Administration (FDA) must show that a supplement is unsafe and causes harm before it can be removed from the market. In 1997, following several hundred reports of adverse effects alleged to be caused by ephedra use, FDA proposed rules to restrict the dosage, require specific warnings on ephedra-containing supplements, prohibit supplements containing ephedrine combined with other known stimulants, and require warnings against excessive intakes.

---

[*] Excerpted from CRS Report RL30750, dated February 4, 2004.

This proposal was criticized for the lack of scientific evidence to support FDA's dosage limitations and the labeling requirements. In 2000, FDA withdrew part of the proposed rule, but subsequent high profile deaths attributed to ephedra led FDA to re-propose the original regulation in 2003. On December 30, 2003, the Department of Health and Human Services (HHS) and FDA announced plans to prohibit sale of ephedra, using the safety provisions of DSHEA for the first time.

Several congressional hearings have focused on the limitations of FDA's current adverse events reporting system, which was used by the agency to conclude that dosage restrictions and mandatory labeling were needed, and specific cases of death attributable to ephedra. A General Accounting Office report examined the scientific basis for FDA's ephedra proposal and concluded that the number of adverse events reports related to ephedra warranted agency attention to safety concerns but failed to provide adequate evidence to support the dosing levels and duration of use limits. In June 2002, HHS announced it would plan expanded research on ephedra's safety, following completion of a RAND Corporation report it had commissioned for review of the existing science. The RAND report indicated that the literature showed that although ephedra can promote a modest short-term weight loss in clinical trials, there is insufficient data on long-term benefits for weight-loss and body building. Combined with other stimulants, it was associated with increased health risks.

In the 108th Congress, H.Con.Res. 52 expresses the sense of the Congress that all major sports organizations should ban the use of ephedra. H.R. 725 would establish labeling and advertising rules for supplements containing ephedra and prohibit sales to minors. H.R. 1025, the Ephedra Public Protection Act, would require pre-market approval for supplements containing ephedra alkaloids and postmarket reporting of serious adverse effects. S.Res. 260 expresses the sense of the Senate that the Secretary of HHS should take action to remove ephedra from the market. These bills were referred to the appropriate committees, but no additional action has yet been taken on any bill or resolution.

BACKGROUND

Ephedrine is the pharmaceutically active compound found in both natural form in herbal ephedra and the synthetic ingredient present in certain over-the-counter (OTC) drug products.[1] Recent attention to the dietary supplements containing ephedra and their regulatory status has been of concern to Congress, the supplement industry and consumers. This report will attempt to clarify the current regulatory status of dietary supplement products containing ephedra.

Ephedra is a botanical, whose herbal properties have been known for centuries by the name of Ma Huang in China, where it was first used as a remedy for the treatment of bronchial asthma. Although some 40 species are known worldwide, its herbal and pharmaceutical effects are attributable to the contents of ephedrine and related alkaloids found primarily in the species of Chinese origin. Historically, practitioners of traditional medicine in China have been trained in the art and skills of compounding small amounts of a variety of botanical ingredients, including ephedra, to treat specific conditions. Ma Huang has generally been consumed in the form of an invigorating tea or infusion with beneficial effects on respiration. Most recently, ephedra in pill form has been promoted for weight reduction and as a performance enhancer in body building and other sports.

In western cultures, ephedrine has been used for years in various drug products. Ephedrine is mainly used as an ingredient in bronchodilator and decongestants, for treating asthma and hayfever, and to combat circulatory collapse in reaction to anesthesia, poisoning, shock and allergic reactions.

The pharmaceutical effects of ephedra are due to the ephedrine alkaloids, but the herbal product may not have the same physiological effect as the pure compound, which can be produced synthetically. The ephedra herb has been used for similar medical purposes, although dietary supplement advocates claim that its action is more gentle and less likely to cause adverse effects. However, a report that investigated the pharmacokinetics of ephedrine from three commercially available herbal Ma Huang products, compared to 25 milligrams (mg) ephedrine hydrochloride capsules showed that the products had similar effect.[2] The authors reported that recent increases in Ma Huang toxicity were not due to the differences in the absorption rates of botanical ephedrine compared with synthetic ephedrine, but instead resulted from accidental overdose often promoted by off-label claims and a belief that natural medicinal agents are inherently safe.

The Dietary Supplement Health and Education Act of 1994 (DSHEA) exempted dietary supplements from the type of premarket approval process that drugs, medical devices and food additives must undergo before they are allowed to be sold. For medical devices and food additives, manufacturers must demonstrate to Food and Drug Administration (FDA) satisfaction that the products are safe through adequate scientific testing prior to marketing. In the case of prescription and OTC drugs, manufacturers must prove, through adequate and well-controlled investigations, that their products are safe and effective before they can be approved for marketing. However, Congress effectively shifted the burden of proof under DSHEA from the manufacturer to the agency to show that a dietary supplement is unsafe, a significantly more difficult standard to meet. Moreover, the agency must demonstrate that the dietary supplement causes harm before it can be removed from the marketplace. In the case of herbal supplements, FDA has only voluntary reports from consumers to rely on, along with generally limited scientific evidence. Very often ephedra is one of several supplements consumers are using, thus complicating a determination of the actual cause of an adverse reaction. Because the law does not require that these products undergo premarket testing and evaluation, there is no reliable baseline information on the possible side effects that can be used to anticipate or compare adverse events. Another confounding factor is research evidence that supplement users are less likely than other consumers to report adverse effects from a product they use.[3]

In contrast, when ephedrine is used in prescription or OTC products, it is regulated as a drug by FDA's Center for Drug Evaluation and Research (CDER). Ephedrine is used for treating mild forms of asthma, and is also approved by the agency for treating such conditions as hypotension, nasal congestion, and sinusitis. FDA considers nonprescription ephedrine to be safe and effective as a bronchodilator, preferably when used under a doctor's care. The dosage recommendations in adults and children over 12 years are 12.5 -25 mg every 4 hours, not to exceed 150 mg per day.[4] According to the industry handbook, the principal adverse effects can include central nervous system (CNS) stimulation, sleeplessness, nausea, loss of appetite, tremors, tachycardia, and urinary retention.[5] The handbook further indicates there are reports that chronic overdose of ephedrine may, in some patients, result in either severe cardiac toxicity or psychosis. Ephedrine, along with other CNS stimulants such as caffeine and phenylpropanolamine, are frequently used as ingredients in products manufactured to physically resemble much stronger controlled substances, such as amphetamines. To prevent both misuse and abuse with the OTC version of ephedrine, an FDA drug advisory committee recommended, and the agency subsequently proposed in 1995 an amendment for more stringent regulation of ephedrine, which is primarily contained in bronchodilators.[6] However, the agency has not finalized the proposed rule on ephedrine in bronchodilators. Denmark, which has considerable research and use experience with ephedrine for weight loss, regulates it as a prescription drug. Recently, the World Health

Organization proposed a restriction on the manufacture and distribution of ephedrinecontaining bronchodilator products.

FDA'S PROPOSAL TO REGULATE HERBAL EPHEDRA

In the 1990s, FDA began receiving reports that consumers were experiencing a variety of adverse effects, allegedly caused by ephedra use. After the agency accumulated several hundred reports of adverse effects, including a number of deaths, attributed to the supplement's use, it convened an ephedra working group, which included members of the FDA Food Advisory Committee and outside experts, on October 11-12, 1995. Following the testimony presented at its first meeting, the group reached no conclusions or determination whether FDA should take any action on regulating these supplements. At a second meeting on August 27-28, 1996, when additional information was reviewed, some group members indicated their concern that there was no safe level of this substance. Others, however, believed that there were certain levels that were safe for use of ephedra.

Subsequently, FDA proposed a rule for ephedra that addressed issues concerning its dosing, labeling and warning statements.[7] The agency proposed that in supplement form a single dose should not exceed 8 milligrams and products should bear required labeling to indicate that no more than 24 mg should be taken in a given day. Also, labeling information was to indicate that the product should not be used for longer than 7 days and required a warning statement that the product was not for long-term use, such as for body building and/or weight loss. The agency also proposed to prohibit the use of ephedra in dietary supplements in combination with ingredients that have a known stimulant effect, such as caffeine, which might cause an interaction. In addition, FDA proposed that a statement accompany any claims that encourage short-term excessive intake to enhance a purported effect, such as increased energy, stating that consuming more than the recommended serving (dose) may result in serious adverse health effects, such as heart attack, stroke, seizure, or death. FDA proposed that these specific warning statements be required to appear on supplement labels when the product contained ephedra.

FDA's proposed regulation generated considerable comment, primarily from consumers and the dietary supplement industry. Most critical comments claimed that FDA's ephedra dosage limitations were not based on scientific evidence, and its labeling requirements were excessive. The voluntary adverse events reporting (AERs) system, which had been the source of the agency's justification for proposing the regulatory changes, also came under scrutiny. The AERs data were criticized for being insufficient to determine whether the adverse events reported were actually caused by ephedra use.

As a result of the continued criticism of the agency's use of the AERs as the basis for its rulemaking, FDA announced in April 2000 that it was withdrawing certain provisions of the proposed rule on ephedra.[8] The provisions that were withdrawn include the dietary ingredient limit for ephedra on a per serving basis, proposed compliance procedures for use of the high performance liquid chromatography method (for sample analysis), limitations on the duration of the product's use, and the prohibition on claims for long-term use, such as for bodybuilding and weight loss. The agency retained the sections of the proposed rule that would prohibit use of ingredients with stimulant effects in combination with supplements containing ephedra, and the requirement that products containing ephedra carry a warning statement on its use by consumers with certain diseases or health conditions or who use certain drugs, accompanied by a recommendation that use be discontinued if they experience certain signs or symptoms.

On March 31, 2000, FDA released 140 additional recent cases of adverse events associated with ephedra use.[9] The agency indicated that these cases had been more fully reviewed and evaluated to determine whether ephedra was the likely cause of the adverse events. FDA also announced its intention to participate in a public forum to address these new adverse events reporting data. At that time, about 1200 cases of adverse events allegedly attributed to ephedra had been reported to the agency.

The Department of Health and Human Service's Office of Women's Health convened the Safety of Dietary Supplements Containing Ephedrine Alkaloids Public Meeting on August 8-9, 2000, to provide an opportunity to review the analysis of adverse events reports by FDA and outside experts. Additional public testimony on recent scientific information on ephedra use was also taken. The *Federal Register* announcement of the meeting sought comments on several questions concerning physiologic actions of ephedra, indications for its use, dosage and duration of use, and risks based on user demographics. It also sought comments on combination use with stimulants, exercise stress and individual sensitivities, and the outcomes associated with dose, user characteristics, and duration of exposure. The meeting revealed the considerable difference of opinion between government and outside reviewers on the evidence concerning the risks associated with using ephedra, based on AERs. Numerous private citizens provided both positive and negative testimonials regarding their personal experience with ephedra use: some reported life-changing weight loss, improvements in other health conditions, and increased energy, while others told of experiencing severe side effects after consuming even minimal doses. Several scientific investigators currently engaged in research on the use of ephedra for weight loss spoke at the meeting, but were unable to disclose the final results of their studies because they had not yet been peer-reviewed and accepted for publication. The summary of the meeting identified several needs: a reliable system for monitoring adverse events; adequate labeling for warnings and contraindications; consumer education; recognition that ephedra use for weight loss and ergogenic purposes constitutes treatment for a health condition (not a dietary supplement structure/function role); long-term trials to establish dose levels and duration guidelines; good manufacturing practices; and a research agenda.[10]

On June 14, 2002, the HHS Secretary Tommy Thompson announced new efforts to expand scientific research on the safety of ephedrine alkaloids and aggressively pursue the illegal marketing of non-herbal synthetic ephedrine alkaloid products.[11] On October 7, 2002, FDA stopped imports of the ephedra-containing products by the Dutch operator selling these products in the United States. In addition, the agency sent inspectors to the New Jersey firm that was distributing the Dutch-made products in this country. When inspectors were denied access to the building, a court order was obtained to enter the building and inspect the company's records. On October 8, 2002, Secretary Thompson announced that he had asked FDA to evaluate the best scientific evidence available and recommend the strongest possible mandatory warning labeling for ephedra-containing products.

Following the deaths of several athletes, FDA reopened for 30 days its earlier proposed rules for ephedra on March 5, 2003. The published document specifically requested comments on the portions of the proposal that addressed dosing, labeling and warning statements, based on new evidence concerning health risks associated with the use of supplements containing ephedrine alkaloids. In addition, the agency signaled its intention to consider whether in light of recent evidence it should determine that ephedra-containing supplements present a "significant or unreasonable risk of illness or injury under conditions of use recommended or suggested in labeling." FDA also sought comments on whether additional legislative authorities would be necessary or appropriate to enable it to address this issue most effectively. The agency had proposed the following warning statement to appear on the principal display panel of the supplement product (see Box 1). The additional information provided in Box 2 was to appear on the outer product label or in product labeling that is an integral part of the outer product packaging, such as information at the point of purchase.

> **Box 1. Proposed Warning Label for Principal Display Panel**
>
> **Warning:** Contains ephedrine alkaloids. Heart attack, stroke, seizure, and death have been reported after consumption of ephedrine alkaloids. Not for pregnant or breast-feeding women or persons under 18. Risk of injury can increase with dose or if used during strenuous exercise or with other products containing stimulants (including caffeine). Do not use with certain medications

On December 30, 2003, HHS and FDA announced plans to prohibit the sale of dietary supplements containing ephedra. The ban will take effect 60 days after the final rule is published. In the meantime, FDA has released a consumer alert that announces its plan to prohibit sales of ephedra-containing dietary supplements and urged consumers to stop using these products. The agency also sent certified letters to over 60 manufacturers who had been producing supplements containing ephedra to provide the companies with advance notice of the final rule to be published to facilitate their earliest compliance. The 60-day period following publication of the final rule is required under the Congressional Review Act. The decision to prohibit the sale of ephedra under the safety provisions of DSHEA represents the first time that the statute has been used to remove a supplement ingredient from the marketplace.

In its announcement of its plans to prohibit the sale of ephedra-containing supplements, the Department indicated that it had reached this decision after conducting an exhaustive and highly resource-intensive process that is required under the provisions of DSHEA for banning a supplement that presents a significant and unreasonable risk to human health. To meet the safety standard, FDA gathered and thoroughly reviewed a prodigious amount of evidence about ephedra's pharmacology, clinical studies of ephedra's safety and effectiveness, newly available adverse events reports, the published literature, and a seminal report by the RAND Corporation. The agency also reviewed tens of thousands of public comments on its February 2003 request for information about ephedra-associated health risks. Coupled with several high-profile deaths alleged to be from ephedra use and the subsequent reopening of the comment period on the previously-published proposed rule on ephedra regulation plus increasing pressure from Congress, the agency's decision is the culmination of a process that began in 1997 when FDA first proposed to require warning statements on the hazards of ephedra use.

Since the announcement on the ephedra ban, the agency has also indicated that it plans to move beyond its recent action against ephedra and increase its focus on certain other supplements. The FDA commissioner recently indicated the agency's intention to examine bitter orange, aristolochic acid and usnic acid, which are ingredients of weight loss products. These three supplement ingredients have been associated with kidney and liver problems.

Box 2. Proposed Additional Information for Product Labeling

This product contains ephedrine alkaloids, which can have potentially dangerous effects on the heart and central nervous system.

Do not use with
a monoamine oxidase inhibitor (MAOI) or for 2 week after stopping a MAOI drug;
certain drugs for depression, psychiatric, or emotional conditions;
drugs for Parkinson's disease;
drugs for obesity or weight control;
methyldopa.

Contact a doctor before using this product if you have or ever had
heart disease, high blood pressure, thyroid disease, seizure, diabetes, depression, and other mental, emotional or behavioral conditions, glaucoma, or difficulty urinating due to prostate enlargement.

Stop use and contact a doctor immediately if these side-effects occur
dizziness, severe headache, rapid and/or irregular heartbeat, chest pain, shortness of breath, nausea, loss of consciousness, or changes in emotions or behavior (such as depression, hallucinations or severe mood swings).

Your risks of serious side-effects from this product can increase
with increased dose, frequency, or duration of use;
if you take it with other dietary supplements containing ephedrine alkaloids (such as ephedra, ma huang, Sida cordifolia);
if you take it with additional products containing stimulants, such as carfeinated beverages and foods (including dietary supplements containing guarana, kola nut, mate yohimbine/yohimbe, Citrus aurantium);
if you take it with medications synephrine, phenylephrine, ephedrine, pseudoephedrine, or phenylpropanolamine;
if you use it before or during strenuous exercise.

CONGRESSIONAL ATTENTION

During a 1999 hearing of the House Committee on Government Reform, the limitations of FDA's current adverse events reporting system were scrutinized.[12] The agency acknowledged that all adverse event reporting cases were posted on its website without being subjected to a vetting process to determine the likely cause of the adverse reaction. According to FDA officials, this process was used to expedite release of adverse cases to interested parties, in lieu of freedom of information procedures which usually take up to a year to respond to specific requests. Thus, the cases are reported as they are received due to the agency's limited resources to review the cases before they are released. Committee members acknowledged that the resources needed to improve the adverse events reporting system were limited.

The House Committee on Science requested that the General Accounting Office (GAO) examine the scientific basis for FDA's ephedra supplement proposal and determine whether the agency adhered to the regulatory flexibility analysis requirements for federal rulemaking. On August 4, 1999, GAO released a report in which it raised concerns about the process by which FDA had compiled the 800 reports on the harmful effects of ephedra.[13] The report indicated that the agency was justified in its determination that the number of adverse events relating to supplements containing ephedra warranted agency attention and consideration of steps to address safety concerns. However, GAO expressed concern about the manner in which FDA used the adverse events reports in supporting the proposed dosing levels and duration of use limits, and concluded that the agency needed additional evidence to support these restrictions. The report indicated that while ephedra might be harmful, the agency lacked adequate data to set dosage levels. GAO concluded that FDA's economic analysis contained the basic elements of a federal agency's cost-benefit analysis; however, the agency analysis was not sufficiently transparent about how it reached its estimate of the costs and benefits of the proposed actions.

In the FY2001 HHS appropriations report (S.Rept. 106-293 accompanying S. 2553), the Senate Committee on Appropriations indicated its continued support for the work of the Office of Dietary Supplements (ODS) at the National Institutes of Health (NIH) and the need for additional research to better inform consumers of the health benefits of supplements. The Committee specifically encouraged ODS to support research on ephedra within the funds provided.

On October 9, 2001, Representative Susan Davis introduced the Ephedrine Alkaloid Consumer Protection Act (H.R. 3066), the first bill to specifically address this dietary supplement ingredient. The bill would have required that supplements containing ephedrine alkaloids be labeled with a warning against use by individuals under 18 years of age, and during pregnancy or nursing. The label would also have directed users to consult a physician before use, if an individual had a personal or family history of a number of health conditions, or if certain drugs or dietary supplement ingredients were being used. The label would also have required a statement that consuming the product might cause adverse health effects, and recommended discontinuing use and contacting a health professional immediately, if certain severe side effects occurred. Labeling would have warned about use of the products when additional caffeine was being consumed, and would have required disclosure of the number of milligrams of ephedrine alkaloids and any other stimulant present in a serving, standardized nomenclature for the ephedrine ingredient, provided a toll-free number and internet address maintained by the Secretary of HHS for reporting adverse effects, a labeling and advertising warning that ephedrine alkaloids were present in the product which may cause adverse health effects and directed the user to read the label and follow directions. The bill would have also prohibited the sale to anyone under the age of 18 years and required ephedrine alkaloid-containing products to be behind the counter in retail establishments. The bill was referred to the House Committee on Energy and Commerce and no additional action occurred.

Several hearings were held in 2002. On July 25, the House Committee on Government Reform convened a hearing on the recent research on the impact of diet and lifestyle on personal health, the growing trend toward obesity and the use of supplements in promoting good health. The draft RAND Corporation report that reviews the literature on health problems associated with ephedra was discussed during the hearing. Subsequently, the Committee requested that GAO review healthrelated calls that one company collected from consumers from May 1997 to July 2002. GAO examined the extent to which consumer information in the records was comprehensive, interpretable and consistently recorded, counted the number of call records reporting types of adverse events that FDA had identified in 1997 as serious or potentially serious, and compared its findings with those of six other reviews of the call records, including one by the company.[14] GAO reported in March 2003 that it counted 96 reports that were for heart attacks, strokes, seizures, deaths and cardiac arrest. The company had identified 78 cases, the other reviews had ranged from 65 to 107 cases.

On July 31, 2002, the Senate Committee on Governmental Affairs' Subcommittee on Government Management, Restructuring and the District of Columbia held a hearing entitled "When Diets Turn Deadly: Consumer Safety and Weight Loss Supplements," which focused on ephedra-containing supplements and the current evidence linking them to serious health problems. Subsequently the subcommittee convened a hearing on October 8, following the death attributed to ephedra of a 16-year-old athlete in the Chairman's district. The hearing focused on the illegal marketing of products containing ephedra to individuals, particularly athletes, in certain age groups. A general consensus of the witnesses was that availability of these products should be restricted for individuals under 18 years of age.

In the 108th Congress, several resolutions and bills that specifically address ephedra/ephedrine alkaloids have been introduced. H.Con.Res. 52 as introduced by Representative Hooley on February 25, 2003, expresses the sense of Congress that all major sports organizations should ban the use of ephedra and dietary supplements containing ephedrine. Currently the National Football League, the National Collegiate Athletic Association, the International Federation of Football Associations and the International Olympic Committee have banned use of ephedra and supplements containing ephedrine. H.Res. 435 was introduced by Representative Davis on November 6, 2003. It expresses the sense of the House of Representatives that the Secretary of Health and Human Services should take immediate action to remove dietary supplements containing ephedrine alkaloids from the market. Both resolutions were referred to the Committee on Energy and Commerce and subsequently to the Subcommittee on Health, but no further action has been taken. S.Res. 260 was introduced by Senator Durbin on November 6, 2003. It expresses the sense of the Senate that the Secretary of Health and Human Services should take action to remove dietary supplements containing ephedrine alkaloids from the market. It was referred to the Committee on Health, Education, Labor, and Pensions, but no further action has been taken.

H.R. 725 was introduced by Representative Susan Davis to amend the Federal Food, Drug and Cosmetic Act to establish labeling and advertising requirements for dietary supplements containing ephedrine alkaloids and prohibit sales to individuals under 18 years of age. The bill would require warning statements and dosage information similar to that proposed by FDA as well as contact information for purposes of the medical product reporting program. In addition to the prohibition of sales to minors, the bill would require that products be held in a portion of the retail establishment not intended to be accessible to its customers. These provisions are similar to the bill introduced in the 107th Congress. The bill was referred to the House Committee on Energy and Commerce and subsequently to the Subcommittee on Health, but no further action has occurred.

On March 4, 2003, H.R. 1025 was introduced by Representative Sweeney, which is entitled the Ephedra Public Protection Act. It would require premarket approval for supplements containing ephedrine group alkaloids and subsequent reporting of serious adverse effects once they were allowed to be marketed. The bill defines 'ephedrine supplements,' 'serious adverse experiences' and 'documented incident.' The bill would also require that the Secretary of HHS publish the proposed rules of good manufacturing practices with 120 days of enactment. (The proposed rules for good manufacturing practices for dietary supplements were actually published on March 13, 2003). Finally, the bill would require the testing of each production lot/batch of ephedrine containing product to ensure label accuracy and carry an expiration date on the label. The bill was referred to the House Committee on Energy and Commerce and subsequently to the Subcommittee on Health, but no further action has yet occurred.

Several days of hearings were convened in 2003. The House Committee on Energy and Commerce held a two-day hearing on issues related to ephedra containing dietary supplements.[15] On the first day, witnesses included victims' families, researchers, several manufacturers, and agency officials. The second day the witnesses included representatives of collegiate and major league sports: baseball, auto racing, football, and soccer. At a hearing convened by the Senate Committee on Commerce, Science, and Transportation on October 28, 2003, the Members heard testimony from representatives of the FDA, the Federal Trade Commission, Anti- Doping Agency, a supplement trade association, consumers, and a scientist. The hearing was designed to determine the availability of supplements to consumers of all ages, industry marketing practices, the effectiveness of DSHEA to protect consumers and whether the current level of domestic consumption exposes consumers to unexpected long- and short-terms effects.

PUBLISHED RESEARCH

On November 6, 2000, the New England Journal of Medicine released an article on the health effects of dietary supplements containing ephedra.[16] The report was the result of an FDA request for an independent review of adverse event reports related to the use of supplements containing ephedra to assess causation, and to estimate the level of risk that use of these supplements poses to consumers. The researchers reviewed 140 reports of adverse events related to ephedra-containing supplements submitted to FDA between June 1, 1997 and March 31, 1999. The results indicated that 31% of cases were considered to be definitely or probably related to the use of ephedra-containing supplements and 31% were deemed to be possibly related. Among the adverse events, 47% involved cardiovascular symptoms (hypertension, palpitations, tachycardia and stroke) and 18% involved the central nervous system (seizures). Ten events resulted in deaths and 13 events produced permanent disability. The authors concluded that the use of ephedra-containing dietary supplements may pose a health risk to some individuals and the findings indicate the need for a better understanding of individual susceptibility to the adverse effects of these supplements. The final version of the report was published in NEJM on December 21, 2000.[17] The early release of the article was a decision of the editors because of the potential public health significance of the study results.

Researchers at several institutions recently conducted a 6-month clinical trial to assess the safety and efficacy for weight loss of an herbal supplement containing Ma Huang and caffeine.[18] They concluded that herbal ephedra and caffeine lowered body weight, fat and BMI (basal metabolic index). Blood pressure was transiently and heart rate persistently increased, but cardiac arrhythmias were not increased. Selfreported symptoms were similar to those for synthetic ephedrine and caffeine products.

A recent report on the use of herbal medicines prior to surgery suggests that certain products may increase the risk of morbidity and mortality.[19] Researchers at the University of Chicago identified eight herbs (including ephedra) that potentially pose the greatest hazard to care of patients undergoing surgery. The study found that, for ephedra, the relevant pharmacological effects included increased heart rate and blood pressure, which increased the risk for heart attack and stroke. Use of the supplement needed to be discontinued at least 24 hours before surgery. The report concluded by suggesting that during the preoperative evaluation, physicians need to explicitly elicit and document a history of herbal medication use, as well as learn the potential preoperative effects of the commonly used herbal medications to prevent, recognize and treat potentially serious problems associated with their use and discontinuation.

A separate analysis of adverse reactions to ephedra and other herbal products during 2001 documented by the Toxic Event Surveillance System was published.[20] Products containing ephedra alone or in combination with other herbs or substances accounted for 64% of all adverse reactions, while these products represented only 0.82% of herbal products sales. The relative risk for an adverse reaction from ephedra was markedly elevated in comparison to all other individual herbs by 10- to 40-fold.

NIH – OFFICE OF DIETARY SUPPLEMENTS

In January 2002, the congressionally mandated Office of Dietary Supplements (ODS) at the National Institutes of Health and the Council for Responsible Nutrition convened a 2-day conference on the science and policy aspects of performanceenhancing supplement ingredients, such as ephedra, androstenedione and creatine. The sessions reviewed the scientific evidence on the benefits and risks of certain supplements in performance enhancement, and the challenges facing regulators, educators and sport health professionals in working with individuals consuming these products.

ODS initiated a systematic review of the literature on ephedra through the Agency for Healthcare Research and Quality (AHRQ), which conducted the analysis in its Evidence-based Practice Center at its RAND-Southern California unit. The review addressed a series of questions related to safety and efficacy of ephedra, alone and in combination with other ingredients, for use in weight management, athletic performance and energy enhancement. The reviewers concluded that ephedrine and ephedra promote a modest short-term weight loss in clinical trials.[21] They determined that there were no data on long-term weight loss, and insufficient evidence to support the use of ephedra for athletic performance. The evidence did show that the use of ephedra or ephedrine with caffeine was associated with increased risk of psychiatric, autonomic or gastrointestinal symptoms, and heart palpitations. The report will be used to assist in shaping the ODS research agenda related to ephedra.

HEALTH CANADA

On June 14, 2001, Health Canada (HC) released an advisory, warning consumers not to use products that contain ephedra, either alone or in combination with caffeine and other stimulants, for weight loss, body building or increased energy.[22] The agency noted that it has authorized ephedrine only for use in nasal decongestants in OTC cold products. Its last action was about 3 years earlier when it addressed Ma Huang use in diet aids. Health Canada had been contemplating issuing the advisory for some time, based on its review of FDA's AER database and 60 AERs, two of which were deaths, related to ephedra use in Canada before October 2000.

In January 2002, Health Canada banned the distribution, sale and/or importation of all ephedra-containing products that had a unit dose of more than 8 milligrams (mg) of ephedra or 32 mg per day, and combination products containing ephedra with other stimulants (such as caffeine). It also banned ephedra products with labeled or implied claims for appetite suppression, weight loss promotion, metabolic enhancement, increased exercise tolerance, body-building effect, euphoria, increased energy or wakefulness or other stimulant effects. Products were to be recalled to the retail level and retailers were to remove the product from store shelves and return them to their suppliers. Health Canada issued this ban under a Class I Health Hazard for a high-risk population (individuals who suffer from certain pre-existing chronic conditions) and a Class II Health Hazard for the general population. Products containing ephedra, which are marketed for traditional medicine, will continue to be available, provided that they do not contain caffeine or exceed the ephedra content of 8 mg per dose to a maximum of 32 mg per day. Products with drug identification numbers that are sold as nasal decongestants and meet the same dose levels will also continue to be available. Health Canada plans to continue to monitor reports of adverse events associated with ephedra and will take further action as necessary. A random market survey was to be conducted within 6 months of the requested recall to determine whether these products have remained off the Canadian market.

STATE REGULATION OF EPHEDRA

In the absence of FDA regulation of dietary supplements containing ephedra, a number of states have attempted to take action to regulate ephedra following reported adverse effects on consumers. State efforts have taken several different forms. Some states have regulated the product by age group, some states have declared it an illegal drug, while other states have adopted regulations on how and to whom it can be sold. See the CRS Congressional Distribution memorandum entitled *Ephedrine: Federal and State Law Regarding Access and Control*, by M. Ann Wolfe and Diana T. Duffy, November 2, 2000, for further information on state action.

In March 2003, Suffolk County, New York banned the sale of ephedra; in April, the New York City Council introduced a bill to ban ephedra sales as well. Subsequently the State of New York banned ephedra sales and California followed suit. Illinois legislation banning the sale of ephedra was signed into law on May 25, 2003, following the death of a 16-year-old high school athlete.

INDUSTRY SELF-REGULATION

Since 1994, the major trade associations representing manufacturers of the dietary supplement industry (the American Herbal Products Association-AHPA, the Consumer Healthcare Products Association-CHPA, the Council for Responsible Nutrition-CRN, the National Nutritional Foods Association-NNFA, and the Utah Natural Products Association-UNPA) have participated in a voluntary program for the formulation and labeling of ephedra-containing products. In many respects, the voluntary program addresses the same issues that were included in the provisions of FDA's proposed rule. The industry's self-regulation provisions were based on the OTC drug standards for ephedrine.

Under the provisions of the voluntary program, a limit on serving size for products containing ephedra is not to exceed 25 mg, for a total of not more than 100 mg per day. Product labeling is required to be in conformity with the standard common name listed in the *Herbs of Commerce*.[23] A listing of the amount of ephedra per serving is required on the label. No synthetically derived ephedrine or their salts are allowed either in the finished product or in raw materials used in their manufacture. Claims that the product may be useful to achieve an altered state of consciousness, euphoria or as a "legal" street drug are not permitted. A label statement including the following information or a statement in conformance with applicable OTC drug monographs must be included:

- Not intended for use by anyone under the age of 18;
- Do not use this product if you are pregnant or nursing;
- Consult a health care professional before using this product if you have heart disease, thyroid disease, diabetes, high blood pressure, a psychiatric condition, difficulty in urinating, prostate enlargement or seizure disorder, if you take monoamine oxidase inhibitor (MAOI) or any other prescription drug, or you are using an over-the-counter drug containing ephedrine, pseudoephedrine or

phenypropanolamine (ingredients found in certain allergy, asthma, cough/cold and weight control products);
- Exceeding recommended serving will not improve results and may cause serious adverse health effects; and
- Discontinue use and call a health care professional immediately, if you experience rapid heart beat, dizziness, severe headache, shortness of breath or other similar symptoms.

Several states have considered, and four (Ohio, Washington, Hawaii and Michigan) have already implemented, adoption of the industry's voluntary standards as their requirements for herbal ephedra products. In May 1999, the supplement industry suggested that FDA adopt the industry's standards either as industry guidance or the basis for developing a regulation.[24] More recently, CHPA has recommended that FDA adopt the industry program standards into regulation.[25]

On October 25, 2000 a citizen's petition on ephedra was filed with FDA by four trade associations (AHPA, CHPA, NNFA, and UNPA).[26] The petition requested that the agency revoke the parts of the 1997 proposed ephedra rule that still stand and implement an industry standard for the labeling and marketing of dietary supplements containing ephedra. The industry standard for labeling and marketing of supplements containing ephedra outlined in the petition are essentially the same as the provisions (outlined above in this report) of the industry's voluntary program that has been in place for more than 8 years. The industry indicated in the petition that virtually all major manufacturers and distributors of ephedra products (represented by the trade associations filing the petition) have already adopted the voluntary program guidelines.

In December 2000, the Council for Responsible Nutrition announced the results of the Cantox Health Sciences International Report that it had funded to review recent clinical trials on the safe use of ephedra.[27] Cantox analyzed in detail 19 clinical trials, AERs from FDA, case reports and published articles, including data from human and animal studies. The report indicated that ephedra is safe to use at a total daily dose of 90 mg, divided into smaller doses of up to 30 mg each, which would cause no observed adverse effects. In addition, a 150 mg total daily dosage was determined to be the lowest level at which moderate adverse effects were first observed.

OBSERVATIONS

The determination by HHS and FDA that ephedra is a risk to public health under the standard for safety in DSHEA represents the first time that the 1994 statute has been used to prohibit the sale of a dietary supplement. The process, which started in 1997, was both time consuming and labor intensive on the part of the Department to establish that it had met the standard of significant and unreasonable risk. The final decision appears to have been based on the collective information available: ephedra's pharmacology, clinical studies of its safety and effectiveness, hundreds of adverse event reports, an extensive review of the published literature, and a report of an independent scientific institute. Assuming that the Department's decision stands up to any challenges that may occur, the ephedra case may serve as a model for the review process and procedures for a supplement that raises public health concern in the future.

The current voluntary adverse reporting system continues to be controversial due to its limitations in providing the information needed to determine causality between the use of supplements containing ephedra and suspected health problems. These limitations have also made it difficult for FDA in its rulemaking to address safety, duration of use and dosage levels for dietary supplements containing ephedra. The AER reports are generally incomplete and difficult to use in establishing whether ephedra was the "cause" of a particular adverse event in a given individual. Furthermore, according to Barnes et al.,[28] the number of adverse reports received into the system may represent an under-reporting of the actual number of adverse events occurring. Future additional research on the use of ephedra for weight reduction may shed some light on its efficacy as well as on any adverse events that may occur in a more controlled research environment and holds out the possibility of evidence of benefits outweighing the risks to the extent that it might be regulated and used as a drug. Congress has also reviewed the problems with the voluntary AERs system for supplements in several hearings and reports and may consider a different means of reporting adverse events for supplements.

Nevertheless, the number of adverse event reports relating to supplements containing ephedra seems to indicate that there is a problem with its use in at least a select group of consumers who experience severe adverse reactions, including lifethreatening events, following use of the supplements. Given the current dearth of controlled clinical trials, it is impossible to ascertain which consumers, many of whom seem to have no known health problems, might be adversely affected by ephedra use. It seems plausible that determining a safe level of ephedra for the general population as a whole may never be possible. In April 2003 the American Heart Association urged a total ban on over-the-counter ephedra sales. The announcement of FDA's decision to prohibit the sale of supplements containing ephedra signals that a final regulation is forthcoming based on the agency's determination at least for now that there is no safe level. However, the final rule will still be subject to the Congressional Review Act, which could alter the final language of the rule.

The congressional language encouraging NIH-ODS to conduct research on ephedra was aimed at helping to generate the answers to numerous questions on the health effects and the vulnerable populations that should avoid use of this supplement. However, no specific funding has been provided for such an initiative; Congress has indicated that it should be supported out of existing funds. While the funding provided to ODS has been increased in recent fiscal years, there are a number of areas of research investigation competing for the monies that the office receives. Furthermore, the results of any research focused on a specific supplement ingredient that is funded by NIH-ODS will not be available for 3-5 years because of the time involved in initiating such a program, completion of the research, and publication of the results in a peer-reviewed journal. Nevertheless, the recent announcement concerning the expansion of research on the safety of these products suggests that the Department recognized the need to seek additional information on the health impact from the use of ephedra-containing supplements. The plans for future research on supplement ingredients may be influenced by the FDA's decision to further examine specific ingredients in dietary supplement products that in its opinion represent potential health problems.

Given the recent high profile deaths associated with ephedra and the amount of controversy surrounding the strict requirements that FDA proposed for dietary supplements containing EA, it will be interesting to see the language of the final rules compared to the original proposed rule. The more moderate voluntary self-regulatory program for the formulation and labeling of ephedra-containing products that the supplement industry has had in place for some time was not adopted by all manufacturers of ephedra-containing products. Bills introduced in the 108th Congress would mandate a number of the provisions of both the FDA proposed rules and the self-regulatory program that the supplement industry has endorsed. Resolution of the regulatory stalemate may have been resolved by the FDA decision to prohibit the sale of this supplement ingredient for now. However, the long-term impact of the ephedra ban may be to raise concern among some lawmakers and others about changes that some believe are needed to make DSHEA more effective in addressing problems in the future.

REFERENCES

[1] Note: Since ephedrine is the active chemical present in both dietary supplements and OTC drug products, the term ephedra will be used to refer to the dietary supplement (natural) form and ephedrine will refer to the drug (synthetic) form for purposes of this report.

[2] Gurley, B., et al. Ephedrine pharmacokinetics after ingestion of nutritional supplements containing *Ephedra sinica* (Ma Huang). Therapeutic Drug Monitoring. 1998. v. 20, pp. 439- 445.

[3] Barnes, J., et al. Different standards for reporting ADRs to herbal remedies and conventional OTC medicines: face-to-face interviews with 515 users of herbal remedies. Journal of Clinical Pharmacology. v. 45, 1998. p. 496-500.

[4] U.S. Department Health and Human Services (HHS). Food and Drug Administration. Cold, cough, allergy bronchodilator, and antiasthmatic drug products for over-the-counter human use. *Federal Register*. v. 56. Apr. 1, 1991. p. 190-197.

[5] American Pharmaceutical Association. Handbook of Nonprescription Drugs. 12th Edition. 1999. Chapter 10. Asthma by D. M. Williams and T. H. Self. p. 229-230.

[6] U.S. Department Health and Human Services (HHS). Food and Drug Administration. *Cold, Cough, Allergy, Bronchodilator, and Antiasthmatic Drug Products for Over-thecounter Human Use.* Proposed Amendment of Monograph for OTC Bronchodilator Drug Products. Notice of proposed rulemaking. *Federal Register* v. 60, no.144. July 27, 1995. p. 38643- 38647.

[7] U.S. Department Health and Human Services (HHS). Food and Drug Administration. *Dietary Supplements Containing Ephedrine Alkaloids.* Proposed rule. *Federal Register* v. 62. June 4, 1997. p. 30678-30724.

[8] U.S. Department of Health and Human Services (HHS). Food and Drug Administration. *Dietary Supplements Containing Ephedrine Alkaloids; Withdrawal in Part.* Proposed Rule. April 3, 2000. *Federal Register* v. 65, no. 64. p. 17474-17477.

[9] U.S. Department of Health and Human Services (HHS). Food and Drug Administration. *Dietary Supplements Containing Ephedrine*

Alkaloids; Availability. Notice. *Federal Register* v. 65, no.64. April 3, 2000. p. 17510-17512.

[10] Jones, W. *Safety of Dietary Supplements Containing Ephedrine Alkaloids.* Public Meeting Aug. 8-9, 2000. Report. 5 p.

[11] U.S. Department of Health and Human Services. HHS Announces Plans To Study Ephedra; Steps Up Enforcement of Illegal Ephedrine Marketing. HHS News. June 14, 2002. [http://www.hhs.gov/news/press/2002pres/20020614.htm]

[12] U.S. House of Representatives. Committee on Government Reform. *How Accurate is the FDA's Monitoring of Supplements Like Ephedra?* 106th Cong., 1st sess. Comm. Print. 106- 60. May 27, 1999. 89 p.

[13] U.S. General Accounting Office. Dietary Supplements: *Uncertainties in Analyses Underlying FDA's Proposed Rule on Ephedrine Alkaloids.* GAO/HEHS/GGD-99-90. July 1999. 79 p.

[14] U.S. General Accounting Office. Dietary Supplements *Review of Health-related Call Records for Users of Metabolife 356.* GAO-03-494. March 2003. 31 p.

[15] House of Representatives. Committee on Energy and Commerce. Subcommittee on Oversight and Investigations, and Commerce, Trade and Protection. Hearings. Issues Relating to Ephedra-Containing Dietary Supplements. July 23 and 24, 2003. 108th Congress, 1st session. Serial no. 108-43. 270 p.

[16] Haller, C. A., and N. L. Benowitz. *Adverse Cardiovascular and Central Nervous System Events Associated with Dietary Supplements Containing Ephedra Alkaloids.* New England Journal of Medicine. Nov. 6, 2000.

[17] Haller, C. A., and N. L. Benowitz. *Adverse Cardiovascular and Central Nervous System Events Associated with Dietary Supplements Containing Ephedra Alkaloids.* New England Journal of Medicine. v. 343, no. 25, Dec. 21, 2000. p 1833-1838.

[18] Boozer, C. N., et al. *Herbal Ephedra/Caffeine for Weight Loss: A 6 Month Safety and Efficacy Trial.* Obesity Research v. 9, no 1. 2001. p. 68.

[19] Ang-lee, M, J. Moss and C. Yuan. *Herbal Medicines and Perioperative Care.* Journal of American Medical Association. July 11, 2001. v. 286, no. 2, p. 208- 216.

[20] Bent, S. et al. *The Relative Safety of Ephedra Compared with Other Herbal Products.* Annals of Internal Medicine. v.138, no.6. Mar. 18, 2003. p.468-471.

[21] Shekelle, P.G. et al. *Efficacy and Safety of Ephedra and Ephedrine for Weight Loss and Athletic Performance.* Journal of the American Medical Association. v. 289, no.12, Mar. 26, 2003 p. 1537-1545.
[22] *Ephedra in Canada.* The Tan Sheet. June 25, 2001. p. 32.
[23] American Herbal Products Association. *Herbs of Commerce.* Austin, Texas, 1992. 78 p. (A compilation of common names of herbs standardized to botanical names in order to reduce nomenclature problems for trade purposes.)
[24] McGuffin, M. American Herbal Products Association. Statement. Presented at the Safety of Dietary Supplements Containing Ephedrine Alkaloids Public Meeting. Aug. 8-9, 2000. 5 p.
[25] Soller, R. W. Consumer Healthcare Products Association. Comments on the safety evaluation of ephedra. Presented at the Safety of Dietary Supplements Containing Ephedrine Alkaloids Public Meeting. Aug. 8-9, 2000. 5p.
[26] APHA, CHPA, NNFA, UNPA. Citizen's Petition to the Food and Drug Administration on Dietary Supplements Containing Ephedrine Alkaloids. Oct. 25, 2000. 6 p.
[27] Cantox Health Sciences International. *Safety Assessment and Determination of a Tolerable Upper Limit for Ephedra.* Dec. 20, 2000.
[28] Barnes, J., et al. *Different Standards for Reporting ADRS to Herbal Remedies and Conventional Otc Medicines: Face-to-face Interviews with 515 Users of Herbal Remedies.* Journal of Clinical Pharmacology. v. 45, 1998. p. 496-500.

INDEX

A

abuse, 11, 17, 22, 23, 31, 43, 49, 58
accuracy, 10, 27, 67
activities, 41, 43, 49
administration, 7, 13, 40, 55, 57, 75, 77
advances, 19
advertising, 56, 65, 66
age, 65, 66, 70, 71
agent, 26
aid, 10, 20, 27
anti-doping policy, 2, 3, 4, 5, 6, 10, 11, 14, 15, 18, 21, 23, 26
association, 3, 4, 10, 12, 13, 16, 20, 22, 24, 25, 30, 38, 39, 43, 44, 49, 67
authority, 9, 30, 38, 40, 49, 50, 51

B

benefits, 20, 56, 64, 69, 73
beverages, 63
bias, 41
business, 44

C

California, 69, 71
Canada, 69, 70, 77
candidates, 41
Caribbean, the, 30
causality, 73
character, 17
children, 42, 43, 58
China, 55, 57
Civic Democratic Party (ODS), 64, 69, 74
classes, 15, 27
Columbia, 34, 66
commitment, 19
community, 27
competition, 5, 6, 15, 18, 19, 27, 30, 42, 44
competitive, 43
compliance, 51, 60, 62
congress, iv, 11, 24, 29, 33, 37, 39, 47, 48, 49, 50, 56, 57, 58, 62, 66, 67, 73, 74, 76
consent, 42
consumers, 57, 58, 59, 60, 62, 64, 65, 67, 68, 69, 70, 73
consumption, 62, 67
contaminants, 28
content, 13, 15, 25, 70
cost-benefit analysis, 64
costs, 64
culture, 42
customers, 66

Customs Service, 40

D

danger, 45
delivery, 27
demographics, 60
Denmark, 58
deterrence, 19
development, 2, 26, 29
disclosure, 65
disease, 27, 63, 71
drugs, 2, 4, 11, 14, 15, 17, 23, 25, 26, 27, 31, 37, 38, 44, 45, 47, 57, 60, 63, 65, 68, 75

E

economic, 64
education, 13, 17, 19, 20, 30, 31, 42, 55, 57, 61, 66
employees, 38, 39, 40, 43
employment, 40, 43
England, 67, 76
English, 35
enlargement, 63, 71
equality, 17, 46
ethics, 17
evaluation, 58, 68, 77
examinations, 38, 44, 46
expectations, 38, 41, 43

F

family, 65
FDA, 55, 57, 58, 59, 60, 61, 62, 63, 64, 65, 66, 67, 70, 72, 73, 74
federal, 11, 15, 22, 23, 31, 38, 39, 41, 44, 49, 53, 64
federal courts, 38, 39
female, 26, 29
firearms, 40
firm, 61

First Amendment, 45
flexibility, 19, 64
food, 57
Fourth Amendment, 40, 41, 43
France, vii, 1, 3
free, 17, 42, 43, 46, 65
freedom, 45, 64
funding, 74
funds, 64, 74

G

Georgia, 41
governance, 43
government, 1, 11, 24, 29, 37, 38, 49, 64, 65, 66, 76
groups, 43, 66
growth, 10, 11, 12, 24, 28, 33, 35
guidelines, 61, 72

H

health, 17, 18, 19, 20, 38, 42, 44, 46, 56, 59, 60, 61, 62, 64, 65, 66, 67, 69, 71, 72, 73, 74
health care, 71, 72
high school, 40, 42, 71
history, vii, 1, 3, 30, 38, 39, 43, 65, 68

I

Illinois, 45, 71
implementation, 2, 4, 41
imports, 61
incentives, 20
incidence, 29
industry, 38, 39, 41, 42, 43, 57, 58, 59, 67, 71, 72, 74
information, 10, 30, 34, 35, 63
inspectors, 61
institutions, 68
integrity, 18, 28, 40, 41, 44
interest, 20, 41, 42, 43, 46

International Olympic Committee (IOC), vii, 1, 3, 30
internet, 65
issues, 49, 59, 67, 71

J

Jones, Bill, 76

L

labeling, 56, 59, 61, 65, 66, 71, 72, 74
labor, 73
language, 15, 74
law enforcement, 40
laws, 17, 45, 49
leadership, 49
learning, 50
legal, iv, 38, 39, 45, 71
legislation, 37, 39, 71
literature, 56, 62, 65, 69, 73

M

Major League Bas, vii, 1, 2, 3, 4, 5, 6, 7, 8, 9, 10, 11, 12, 13, 14, 15, 16, 17, 18, 20, 21, 22, 23, 24, 25, 26, 32, 33, 39, 48
Major League Baseball Players Association (MLBPA), 3, 5, 6, 7, 8, 9
male(s), 26, 28, 29
management, 5, 10, 27, 44, 66, 69
manufacturing, 61, 67
market, 55, 56, 66, 70
marketing, 57, 61, 66, 67, 72
measures, 39
Mexico, vii, 1, 3
minors, 56, 66
model, 18
monitoring, 61
movement, vii, 1, 2, 3, 4, 15, 18, 20, 30

N

national, 40
National Basketball Association (NBA), vii, 1, 5, 6, 7, 8, 9
National Football League (NFL), vii, 1, 3, 5, 6, 7, 8, 9

O

ODS, see Civic Democratic Party, 64, 69, 74
Olympics, 5, vii, 1, 4, 5, 11, 15, 24, 52
organization(s), vii, 1, 4, 5, 10, 12, 13, 16, 17, 18, 20, 21, 28, 31, 56, 66

P

parents, 42
penalties, 14, 15, 39, 48, 50, 52
performance, vii, 1, 3, 4, 16, 27, 28, 37, 38, 40, 47, 49, 50, 55, 57, 60, 69
performance-enhancing substances, vii, 1, 3, 4, 16, 40, 49, 50
permit, 40
policy(ies), vii, 1, 2, 3, 4, 5, 6, 7, 8, 9, 10, 11, 12, 14, 15, 16, 17, 18, 19, 20, 21, 22, 23, 25, 32, 33, 37, 39, 42, 43, 46, 47, 48, 49, 50, 52, 55, 69
population, 70, 74
power, 27, 45
prejudice, 45
primary, 41
principal, 62
private sector, 38, 40
procedures, 38, 40, 43, 45, 47, 48, 49, 50, 51, 53, 60, 64, 73
production, 27, 28, 67
programs, 13, 18, 31, 37, 39, 45, 48
promote, 17, 26, 46, 56, 69
public health, 68, 73
public policy, 3

R

raw materials, 71
regulation(s), 35, 38, 39, 40, 41, 42, 44, 49, 50, 53, 56, 58, 59, 62, 70, 71, 72, 74
regulators, 69
religion, 45
report, vii, 1, 2, 3, 4, 16, 40, 47, 48, 49, 50, 56, 57, 58, 62, 64, 65, 67, 68, 69, 72, 73, 75
research, 18, 19, 20, 29, 30, 44, 56, 58, 61, 64, 65, 69, 73, 74
responsibility, 25
retail, 65, 66, 70
revenue, 32, 41, 46
risk(s), 19, 20, 43, 56, 60, 61, 62, 63, 68, 69, 70, 73

S

safety, 11, 23, 31, 38, 40, 42, 43, 44, 46, 56, 61, 62, 64, 68, 69, 73, 74, 77
sample, 27
science, 19, 56, 69
secondary, 29
security, 40
self, 17, 43, 44, 71, 74
self-regulation, 71
Senate, 18, 19, 32, 33, 56, 64, 66, 67
skills, 57
standards, 2, 38, 39, 40, 44, 45, 48, 49, 71, 72, 75
steroids, 2, 3, 5, 7, 8, 10, 11, 14, 16, 17, 20, 22, 23, 24, 25, 26, 28, 29, 33, 37, 38, 44, 45
study, 50, 68

summaries, 39
supervision, 11, 23, 31
suppliers, 70
Supreme Court, 40, 41, 42
survey, 23

T

telephone, 10
Texas, 77
threshold, 27, 43
threshold level, 43
trade, 50, 67, 71, 72, 77
training, 3
transport, 27

U

U.S. Anti-Doping Agency (USADA), 4, 30
United States (US), vii, 1, 3, 9, 11, 16, 20, 23, 31, 33, 35, 39, 48, 49, 61

W

water, 27, 29
welfare, 43
White, 32
women, 62
work, 19, 43, 64
workers, 38, 39, 40, 44
World Anti-Doping Agency (WADA), 2, 4, 30, 50